Breakthrough

Breakthrough:

The Psilocybin School

Grant Cameron

First Printing March 2021
ISBN: 9798713113100

Itsallconnected Publishing
whitehouseufo@gmail.com
www.itsallconnected.weebly.com
www.presidentialufo.com

Surrender is the only rule
Believe me
Surrender is the only rule

Contents

DISCLAIMER

May these sacred plants provide illumination on your journey and bring you closer to the god within you.

All chemical experimentation described in this book was conducted under medical supervision in a safe and controlled environment.

Please check your local regulations/laws thoroughly before purchasing any chemicals mentioned in this book. Only purchase from reputable, legal distributors.

Each individual will react to these chemicals differently. Dosages, frequency, and side effects will be unique to the user. As such attempting to follow the dosages mentioned in this book is not recommended.

I do not advise nor recommend the recreational use of the chemicals mentioned in this book. If you are considering taking any chemicals not already prescribed to yourself, it is recommended you first consult a medical professional.

Introduction

What I want to underscore is that what I am about to write is just a story. We so poorly understand consciousness. I think psychedelics are unique in their capacity to shine a bright light on what it is to be aware – what it is to be conscious. If you think about that, that is a very profound thing called the hard problem of consciousness. The hard problem is that it may not be reduceable to reductionistic neuroscience. It is an open problem philosophically and scientifically, although my materialistic-oriented colleagues from the sciences might push back on that. They would strongly think of consciousness as an epiphenomenon of the brain network function...right now, it does not seem to be solvable.

-Roland Griffiths, American psychopharmacologist. He is a professor of neuroscience, psychiatry, and behavioral science, and director of the Center for Psychedelic and Consciousness Research at Johns Hopkins University School of Medicine

The Universe does not exist "out there," independent of us. We are inescapably involved in bringing about that which appears to be happening. We are not only observers. We are participators. In some strange sense, this is a participatory universe. Physics is no longer satisfied with insights only into particles, fields of force, into geometry, or even into time and space. Today we demand of physics some understanding of existence itself.
-Physics Nobel Laureate John Wheeler

Eventually, even Pavlov found that when he heard a bell, he had the overwhelming urge to feed a dog.
-AainaA-Ridtz

This is the third book in which I have written about the subject of psilocybin. Psilocybin is a naturally occurring tryptamine alkaloid in what is known as "magic mushrooms." It's the principal psychoactive component of the Psilocybin genus of these mushrooms.

This book contains my experiences during my controlled experiments consuming psychedelic mushrooms. It is merely a journal of my encounters that I feel I have now deciphered. Since the experiments, I have integrated them into my daily life, and now I understand how they might fit into ultimate reality.

Some speak about magic mushrooms as either an insane, delusional drug, a great gift of the Gods, or a trap by the devil to capture our souls into an eternal hell.

I have never done drugs in my life, even though I lived through the 1960s era of social, musical, and artistic change heavily influenced by psychedelic drugs. I have recently been interested in psilocybin because it appeared to be a contact modality that I could employ to get into "the field." In my book, *Contact Modalities: The Keys to the Universe*, we discuss these 'modalities' as being different ways to access the elusive, invisible "field." Many people have reported accessing this "field." It is a state of mind, perhaps, and a place where people report receiving messages from the Universe, gaining inspiration or downloads, witnessing paranormal events or experiences, having intuitive insights or telepathy with other beings. It is a way to connect to people like deceased relatives or aliens through activities such as CE-5.

My past inexperience allowed me to bring clear sight to the modern explorations in psychedelics. I also came in without any medical memberships in which psilocybin might pad the bottom line. Lastly, I do not have any membership in any psychedelic organization that needs to be vindicated.

In the 16 sessions shared with the reader in this book, I discovered that ideas and sensed images would appear in my mind's eye when my eyes were closed. I have never had anything like this occur during my meditations, and there have been many of them.

From these 16 sessions, I developed a protocol that seems predictable, safe, and was successful for me in producing the material that appeared in my mind's eye. Every session I experienced brought with it a different lesson, and I merely audio recorded in real-time what I sensed and then documented the material on paper.

Conditioned Mind

Science cannot long remain unfettered in a social system that seeks to exercise control over the whole spiritual and intellectual life of a nation. The correctness of a scientific theory can never be adjudged by its readiness to give the answers desired by political leadership.
-Charles A. Leone

Psilocybin, from what I have researched, and discovered through personal experience, is nothing more than a contact modality. It takes an individual into an altered state, a higher vibrating state, or a more fluid state outside the belief structure that makes up our everyday waking reality. Another way to put it is that psilocybin is the portal to extended consciousness found not *out there* but within ourselves.

The situation is similar to what people experience when they put on their glasses as they get out of bed. Those glasses make them see things that would otherwise be invisible. It is the same world seen through a filter or opening that exposes a new reality.

Another analogy would be the video games played by millions every day. There are multiple levels within each game, which are only accessible by learning how to get into the more complex level. Most people believing in physical reality are stuck playing only on the first, most superficial level of the video game.

That state may contain information that will help one break out of the conditioned mind, which dictates how we see the world around us. It comes from all the ideas taught to us in the early years of our life, which become our concrete notions about the world.

Through our cultural norms, I am asked to believe that I am a Caucasian male, a Canadian, middle class, that there are enemies around the world that I should fear, and that there is a God who demands we do certain things in our life. We take on these beliefs from those around us and adopt them as our own; if we evaluated them before accepting them, or worse yet, that we independently thought them up ourselves, then we could become victims of these outside ideas.

If I were born in China, I would not be speaking English or singing "God Bless America." If I were born in an Arab country, I might view the Western world as the Great Satan. I would not worship the same God nor eat the same food.

The conditioned mind extends into how we understand reality as well. At one time in recent history, we were told that: the world is flat, the sun revolves around the world, we are at the center of the Universe, we are alone in the Universe, matter is solid, dreams are hallucinations, everything is happening by accident, everything we see accidentally came from nothing for no particular reasons, and that the human nervous system cannot safely control automobiles at speeds faster than horses can gallop.

These outside ideas are not our own, but we cycle them through the basal ganglia in the brain, where they become habits and patterns. What is beyond the conditioned mind? Where do we tap into *true* reality? How do we change the conditioned mind programmed in childhood?

Rebecca Gladding, M.D., a clinical instructor and attending psychiatrist at UCLA, stated that the conditioned mind comprises a "series of deceptive brain messages, society's rules, and parent's expectations. They are things that are conditioned."

Nobel Laureate Max Planck stated, "A new scientific truth does not triumph by convincing its opponents and making them see the light, but rather because its opponents eventually die and a new generation grows up that is familiar with it."

Planck would indicate there is nothing except death that changes the conditioned mind. However, Psychedelics research strongly suggests that the conditioned mind can be changed entirely, and the brain can be rewired with new and more accurate reality concepts.

Psychotherapist Ralph Metzner stated that psychedelics have a great power to change the conditioned mind to a "true self" state that existed before somebody programmed the conditioned mind. Still, the intention going into a session with psychedelics would determine if the old conditioning gets replaced with positive or negative new concepts:

> *Psychedelics don't really do anything. The question is, what do you want to do? What does a person want to do when taking a psychedelic? What is the intention? That's what this 'set and setting' gets at, which was Leary's invention. The set or intention is the most important thing because the set determines the intention. The best definition of a psychedelic is that they are 'non-specific awareness amplifiers...'*
>
> *Charles Manson gave his acolytes LSD to create death and mayhem. It was not a consciousness-expansion experience. The CIA, that was the first to research with psychedelics. They used it in order to confuse people. They thought they could confuse the enemy, so they won't know what they are doing. We will slip it to people, and they will do crazy things. It is indiscriminate. It is a tool, a non-specific awareness amplifier.*[1]

The "set and setting" is a common idea amongst the psychedelic community. It refers to the mindset (set) of the person going into the trip. The setting is the environment that you are in, be it your bedroom or a park. Tim Leary actively researched whether having a conducive, comfortable setting and a loving, open mindset would induce a good trip. In contrast, a bad trip might be provoked when being in a fearful headspace or a public, chaotic environment. Leary said:

> *Of course, the drug dose does not produce the transcendent experience. It merely acts as a chemical key — it opens the mind, frees the nervous system of*

its ordinary patterns and structures. The nature of the experience depends almost entirely on set and setting. Set denotes the preparation of the individual, including his personality structure and his mood at the time. Setting is physical — the weather, the room's atmosphere; social — feelings of persons present towards one another; and cultural — prevailing views as to what is real. It is for this reason that manuals or guide-books are necessary. Their purpose is to enable a person to understand the new realities of the expanded consciousness, to serve as road maps for new interior territories which modern science has made accessible.[2]

My role in experimenting with psilocybin was to be a noetic explorer, seeking information not obtainable using just the conscious ego-mind. I was not interested in becoming a therapist or a marketer of the substance, but someone looking into how the psilocybin experience could explain ultimate reality.

My psilocybin study was part of a more significant inter-disciplinary research that involved other Contact Modalities such as meditation, yoga, hypnosis, holotropic breathing, and brain injury, which have been shown to lead people into similar states of non-local mind, which is unbounded in space and time.

My research linked into the group of drugs known as psychedelics, which affect the serotonin 5-HT2A receptor. Science will reference this receptor as the basis of the chemistry that causes people's "hallucinations." However, this is short of the truth.

In reality, all psychedelics affect the serotonin 5-HT2A receptor, but each of the drugs: psilocybin, LSD, DMT, and 5-MeO-DMT, all produce entirely different experiences. Therefore, it proves that there is much more going on beyond some molecule getting locked into a receptor.

The first kind of mushrooms I took was called *Golden Teachers*. I felt this was appropriate because I wanted to go into the experience to learn something. I suspect that it is the more extroverted person who would be interested in a psilocybin trip with a group of people at a concert, at a party, or in an outdoor gathering. However, I intended my introverted self to be learning lessons alone as if I was going to school.

The idea goes back to when humanity believed that the Earth was flat. The rational, analytic Scientific minds at the time had observed, measured, and determined that the world was flat. It made total sense! If it were not, all the water would run off the ball, and people on the bottom of the Earth would fall off.

The people of the day just recycled the same ideas over and over. Without new evidence, there was no reason to change the belief. Changing beliefs come from new experiences - whether that be a personal experience or an experiment in a lab. It was not until Christopher Columbus provided the unique experience of sailing west from Spain and not falling off the Earth's edge that people started to consider the flat-Earth idea might be incorrect. A new and expanded worldview had begun.

Even then, like any new idea introduced into the world, the skeptics scoffed at the latest evidence, and it took many years for the paradigm to change. Some have not transformed thinking even today as many holds to the flat Earth theory.

In my book called *Contact Modalities: The Keys to the Universe*, I discuss many modalities that brought in new information to challenge the idea that the physical 3D world is all there is.

By trying the psilocybin modality, I imagined I could bring some new ideas into my mistaken worldview. And then I could share them with others.

I decided to begin my trips at particular times so that I can go about my regular timetable the following day; these times would be either 8:00 pm or 3:00 am. I would tell myself that it was time for school, time for the lessons to begin. My intention was that I was going to access the "field" and get some instruction that I could not obtain in the regular 3D world.

I received a different lesson in each session. I was not surprised when the experience changed; I knew with the opening scene precisely what the lesson would be and what I would be dealing with.

On Memory

Most of my sessions were audio-recorded and transcribed. The recordings provided many benefits over merely reflecting on the session after it was over.

Once starting a session, I would instruct myself to "own it." That helped take the fear away, as it removed me as a victim and made me an observer of what would happen. I took responsibility for what circuitry in my brain that I purposely exercise and stimulate. Once I accepted responsibility and removed myself from being a victim, it worked quite well.

People believe in Darwin's theory of survival of the fittest. This has created a world view of victimhood where we are fearful and unhappy because we have been dealt a bad hand in life. We accept the notion that we are missing what will make us happy.

For myself, I could say that if I didn't live in Winnipeg (the coldest major city in the world), I would be happy. If I lived more in nature instead of in a city, then I would be satisfied. If I had money, life would be more comfortable. If I had loving relatives, then I would be content. If I had a good job that I liked, happiness would ensue, and on and on.

Owning it changes all that. It is possible to be happy and fulfilled wherever I live whether I have no money, no loving relatives, or a good job. All that is necessary is to accept the experience. It is all a matter of our belief system, and as physicist Nobel Laureate John Wheeler says, it is a participatory universe. What you bring into a situation with your thoughts is what you will manifest and make happen. There may be no event without the participant. Moreover, Wheeler stated, "there is no out there, out there," so it may all be one internal experience.

In the UFO world, there is an analogy to the idea that there is nothing outside of ourselves. Emmy award-winning investigator, George Knapp, talked about what he had observed in the famous Skinwalker Ranch investigation in Utah. He stated that those who were the most aggressive and emotional when seeing the phenomena had the worst experiences because of their connection to it via their emotional interactions.

The same idea occurs in the worldview of reincarnation. We come into the world to experience things, and we choose subconsciously, if not consciously, what the lessons and experiences will be. Therefore, we *chose* what is happening to us right now. We have to own the fact that we came into this world at this particular time and place, in the middle of whatever utopia or nightmare we are experiencing. Instead of playing the victim and blaming outside forces for our state of mind, we must take responsibility for what happens. It is only an *us vs. them* world if you see it that way.

Similarly, when a person goes under hypnosis and faces a challenging memory, hypnotists can suggest that the person holds a balloon to remove themselves from the scene so they can view it as an observer.

My experience with my psilocybin sessions is that they were all very fluid and meaningful. Still, the minute the incident was over, my memory of the session would start to fade as quickly as a dream upon awakening.

My perception is that the left brain is being quieted just as in hypnosis, meditation, holotropic breathwork, or inside of a dream. These non-ordinary states of consciousness and shamanic instructions are only presented in images translated in the right-brain. There is no left-brain voice. There were no left-brain written instructions.

The minute I came out of the psilocybin state, the left brain came back online, and the experience faded like a dream upon awakening. Luckily, I audio-recorded while the session was going on.

Facts and Belief

Modern science is based on the principle: 'Give us one free miracle, and we'll explain the rest.' The one free miracle is the appearance of all the mass and energy in the Universe and all the laws that govern it in a single instant from nothing. This notion is the limit case for credulity. In other words, if you can believe this, you can believe anything."
-Terence McKenna

I have never run into anything evil with a capital E. The difficult thing that I have run into is stuff out of my own stack. That is the best way that I can put it. I am not saying that cannot exist by that is not something that I have run into...now I have run into saints, spirit guides, golden presences, and sources of light. Those are all great, and I have run into those a lot.
-Kara, who had hundreds of high-dose psychedelic experiences

All the belief in the world and fifty cents will not buy you a cup of coffee. Although most people trust their opinions implicitly, they will declare "I believe this" and "I don't believe that." The person beside them may have precisely the opposite beliefs and be just as assured that he is right.

How then do we discover the truth? It may be through accessing noetic material. Many of the significant discoveries and inventions in history have come through accessing noetic information. That is where contact modalities come in. They are the gateway to the inner essence of our thoughts.

People think that there are hard facts that make up their concept of the world. I believe that a closer look will show that everything is only a belief—both science and religion claim to be proving things. In our recent past, we were told to follow what the ministers said, and now We set up our belief system based on new theories that science proposes. "Science Sunday School" is the marriage of these two false belief systems where "we know, and you just believe."

As mentioned above, people see things through filters which are similar to glasses. We get so used to what we see we forget that we are wearing the glasses that distort it.

A second more dramatic example of this is the experiment done by psychologist George Stratton, who wore specialized glasses that turned his vision upside down for eight days. By the third day, he saw the world entirely as usual -- as if he was not wearing the glasses. When he then took the glasses off, he saw everything upside down for a while. In each case, the mind flipped the upside-down image that it was receiving and corrected it. Seeing is not believing.

That is why people in the United States can be so divided in politics. Half of the population thinks that President Trump is a brilliant genius and will make the country great again. The other half thinks he is foolish and has destroyed the country. If the process were rational and analytical, everyone would come to the same conclusion. These examples show us that if we attach ourselves to either one belief or its opposite, we do not see the complete picture. To do that, as in good journalism, one must know both points of view. Then we can take the truth out of each and choose one in the middle, where we can be more objective and less emotional with fewer filters that distort the truth.

The father of American psychology, William James, who explored the intersections of science and mysticism, was one of the first to point out the fallacy of such "we've proved it" thinking. He stated, "A great many people think they are thinking when they are merely rearranging their prejudices."

Much of this confusion of proof versus belief comes from the rational, analytical, left-brain, and the left-brain interpreter, which also resides in that side of the brain. The left brain is skeptical and cynical about what it sees around it. It is always alerting the individual to be wary of the things it sees around. It presents its conclusion as logic analysis versus just subjective belief. It fails to consider that the logical proof it claims to hold will be nonsense in 100 years and is merely a belief.

Albert Einstein considered David Bohm to be his intellectual successor. Like Bohm, Einstein realized that there was a problem with assuming too many things regarding knowledge. He expressed this by saying, "We can't solve problems by using the same kind of thinking we used when we created them."

A closer look indicates that the way we solve problems involves nothing more than recycling the same ideas, just like shuffling around chairs on the deck of the sinking Titanic. We fail to recognize the power of belief and how easily we adopt opinions as opposed to facts.

That is where psilocybin and other contact modalities come in. Psilocybin is one of many contact modalities that allows individuals to get into a field of knowledge that appears to contain new ideas, new thinking, and new deck chairs, and if William James is correct, "insight into depths of truth."

The Noetic Flow State

> No•et•ic: *From the Greek noēsis/ noētikos, meaning inner wisdom, direct knowing, intuition, or implicit understanding.*

This noetic flow state brings in the information that comes with absolute certainty. That field is where the word noetic comes from. The data retrieved by the flow state is viewed, as William James described it, as:

...states of knowledge. They are states of insight into depths of truth unplumbed by the discursive intellect. They are illuminations, revelations, full of significance and importance, all inarticulate though they remain, and as a rule, they carry with them a curious sense of authority for after-time.

I have had several noetic experiences. One occurred in 2012 and the other in 2017. None of the material that I received in either session turned out to be wrong. Much of the information has been supported, such as the experience in 2012 where I got the idea that consciousness was at the basis of the UFO problem. In 2012, a handful of people believed this, but now in 2020, it is a common conversation topic.

The best analogy to understand this is Michael Pollan's account about interviewing patients involved in the smoking sensation program at Johns Hopkins University using high-dose psilocybin. The program has an 80% success ratio after one year with people who were lifelong smokers. This compares with other methods like the patch, which is 20% or less effective or talk therapy with a success ratio of about 2%. So, what is the difference?

As a lifelong smoker, I know that whatever they were using must have power not found in this 3D world. It turns out that the key is the noetic quality (embedded in the mind as revealed truth or actual knowledge) of the experience. Rather than seeing commercials that make you afraid and hearing how bad smoking is, one woman described how she went from a lifelong smoker to a non-smoker, using nothing but a five-hour psilocybin session with integration counseling. Pollan asked one woman how she managed to stop smoking:

> *I remember there was this Irish woman, about 60, and she said, 'well, I had this incredible experience. I sprouted wings and flew all through European history, and I saw all these great scenes in European history. I died three times, and I saw my ashes, my smoke rise from my body on the Ganges River. I realized that, God, there is so much to do and see in the world that killing yourself with cigarettes is really stupid.' She knew that, and people had probably told her that before, but now she believed it.[3]*

More importantly, there are ineffable, indescribable characteristics of mystical information received while using psilocybin. There are no words in the English language to describe what is being seen and felt. This causes trouble with university psychedelic researchers in that they have never had the experience themselves. It does not stop some from stating that the subjects are framing what they are experiencing, implying that it is just an experience and they as researchers can sort the wheat from the chaff. In this manuscript, I have stated that this is a bit like the Pope talking about different sex techniques or giving marriage counseling advice.

In 2017, I had a noetic flow-state experience that spoke to this. I was told during this experience that humans confuse knowing and believing. We think we know when we just believe. This happens with scientists who believe they can sit on the outside and evaluate the anecdotal stories. They think they know, but they have not got a bloody clue. (This same message was also given to me as a download in Session #7 and #8 in this book)

The researchers have little understanding because what happened was beyond words, and they were not there. Therefore, they can only believe based on what they were taught in "Science Sunday School" over the years.

Some scientists have it entirely backward (which was my basic message in 2017). The ones who take the psilocybin have the experience of "insight into depths of truth unplumbed by the discursive intellect," but not the researcher. He just believes that he knows. If anyone has had a glimpse of true reality, it is the psilocybin subject. They know, and the researcher just believes.

The skeptic will still say they don't believe it, which is fine. Just keep the emphasis on the word *belief* because that is all it is, and one dollar and all the belief in the world will not buy a cup of coffee.

We have belief on one side and noetic material on the other side. I think the money is better spent studying the noetic material, as everyone who experiences it has a *knowing* which to them represents the REAL reality. I believe the 3D world is just a world based on psychosis and mistaken beliefs, but the *knowing* these people get represents actual reality. Their noetic experiences are almost always reported and contain the idea that everything is one and everything is conscious.

One collection of evidence that shows a noetic field exists, and how precise and accurate it is, is all the inventions that came noetically, where the scientist or inventor described that the invention or discovery just popped into his/her head. Along with that came the certainty that the material was a glimpse into a different reality that they had to pursue.

The book I wrote called, *Inspired: The Paranormal World of Creativity,* described many of the most significant inventions and discoveries of all times. In each of the ones researched, the person knew with certainty that they had arrived at the answer. Reportedly Einstein said, "I knew I had to understand that dream, and you could say, and I would say, that my entire scientific career has been a meditation on my dream." Larry Page, who had a dream that led him to create Google, also talked about how quickly he acted on the dream, "I grabbed a piece of paper and started writing."

Here are some examples of information received as a download:

Inventor	Discovery	Method
Albert Einstein	Theory of Relativity	Dream
Nicola Tesla	Alternating Motor	Sudden insight
Niels Bohr	Quantum Atom	Dream
Larry Page	Google	Dream
Charles Towns	Laser	Sitting on park bench
Dennis Gabor	Hologram	Waiting to play tennis.
Elias Howe	Sewing machine	Dream
Dimitry Mendeleev	Periodic Table	Dream

Dr. Jim Fadiman, a psychologist, described how early LSD research used this understanding to its advantage to solve 40 or 44 challenging problems in minutes:

We brought in senior scientists from a number of the local industries that were developing a lot of different products. And we also brought in some professors who were doing theoretical research, so we had problems ranging from NOR Gate Theory, which is an abstract mathematical area used in circuit design, to space probes, for solar properties, microtome, improvements in tape recording technology. We also had some architects, and we said we want projects that your clients have consistently already turned you down with.

(After taking) One dose. They were given three to four hours basically of intense work. The comments

from a number of them are the work is not noticeably better than their own good work, but instead of weeks, it was minutes. And that, of course, was extraordinary in its own right. And the other side of it is that we asked them, several months later, had there been any residual creative effect? And what they said is, "Yes." Up to several months, and we didn't really ask beyond that, they had increased creativity, slowly diminishing back to their baseline. And the main way they were more creative is they were more focused; they were able to let go of solutions that weren't working. And the other thing, and this is peculiar to psychedelic, they were much more easily able to see patterns that they had not noticed before. So many of them said, "I suddenly was able to take a totally new approach.4

The psychedelic or mystical state also comes with absolute certainty. That was one of the things that I noticed in many of my psychedelic sessions. It was not just "this is a good idea" but "this is the answer!" This certainty is a concept that is incomprehensible to those who have not experienced it. It will not change the mind of most scientists who would claim that the dream is subjective and that they know more about the dream than the subject who had the dream.

Despite all these, many skeptics who have not had a high-dose psilocybin session will remain unconvinced. That is because they have come into the research discussion with a preconceived belief that interferes with their ability to make an independent assessment of the data. Without new data, scientists are merely recycling the same ideas that created the old paradigm.

The old paradigms created by the rational, analytical mind generated ideas like the flat earth, the geocentric model, the atom being indivisible, there is only one galaxy, and the notion that we are the only intelligent life in the Universe will remain in place until new, conflicting information is introduced.

Scientists often state that they are skeptical but open-minded or that because they are "scientific," their materialistic worldview is proven fact. Therefore, any extraordinary psilocybin claims that make the nuts and bolts' view of the world unstable will require extraordinary evidence to change their belief paradigm (which they would describe as knowledge paradigm.)

Most will unconsciously take the position like that of eminent physicist Albert Michelson, who said in 1894: "it seems probable that most of the grand underlying principles have been firmly established and that further advances are to be sought chiefly in the rigorous application of these principles to all the phenomena which come under our notice...the future truths of physical science are to be looked for in the sixth place of decimals."

The fact is that science's belief structure is often overrun by assumptions and faith. They may acknowledge these issues but claim it will not influence them because they are open-minded. This is like saying a person is an alcoholic but can be detached while working in a brewery.

The psychedelic research must be managed with proper research protocols. There may be a new finding that appears and seems contradictory. It must be investigated. The researcher's conscious mind looks at it and creates a hypothesis as to what it might be. Experiments are then run to test the theory.

When the experiments are completed, observations as to what happened are made, and a conclusion is reached to see if the issue was what it appeared to be or if it is something else.

If it is something else, then new experiments are run to test that hypothesis, and more observations are made as to what materialized. That leads to new conclusions, which engenders new experiments, observations, and findings. Each cycle brings the researcher closer to what true reality is.

Understanding true reality is like a chess game where the opponent is neither good nor bad. The game's goal is to figure out why the opponent moved a particular piece, and then that action can give a hint of what countermove can be made to win.

Every time the opponent moves a piece, we must objectively determine why that piece was moved and how it fits into the overall game.

Mystical Experience

[Noetic refers to] states of insight into depths of truth unplumbed by the discursive intellect. They are illuminations, revelations, full of significance and importance, all inarticulate though they remain, and as a rule, they carry with them a curious sense of authority...
-William James, philosopher

The modern study of the mystical experience began with William James, who issued a highly influential, two-volume synthesis and summary of psychology in 1890, Principles of Psychology. He also offered the first course in psychology.
-William James described the mystical experience in his famous collection of lectures published in 1902 as "The Varieties of Religious Experience"

I n his research and writing, the late writer Aldous Huxley wrote that the conscious mind effectively was a reducing valve that filtered out a good percentage of things in reality. He wrote:

To make biological survival possible, Mind at Large has to be funneled through the reducing valve of the brain and nervous system. What comes out at the other end is a measly trickle of the kind of consciousness which will help us to stay alive on the surface of this particular planet.

After Huxley, many others have spoken of psychedelics as a gateway to open up a valve and allow all manner of transpersonal experiences from the rest of reality to flow in.

One of the key elements that have been reported across the board through psychedelics (and other non-drug modalities) is a report of what has come to be called 'the mystical experience.' These are its criteria:

1. **Conscious Unity**-The boundaries of where you perceive your individual identity to begin and end ultimately vanish (otherwise known as ego death). Instead, you are left with a boundless and infinite union with all that is around you.

2. **No Time or Space**-Rather than seeing past and future, everything becomes a series of eternal 'now moments.' Without time, space is endless.

3. **Objective Reality or Noetic[1] Quality**- The experience comes with absolute certainty that what you are experiencing is profound reality instead of a good idea. Everything seems perfect, and every event has a purpose. William James said, "They are states of insight into depths of truth unplumbed by the discursive intellect. They are illuminations, revelations, full of significance and importance, all inarticulate though they remain; and as a rule, they carry with them a curious sense of authority for after-time."

---

[1] no•et•ic: From the Greek noēsis/ noētikos, meaning inner wisdom, direct knowing, intuition, or implicit understanding.

4. **Gratitude**-The experience comes with an enormous state of gratitude. The vastness and grandeur of the Universe become apparent. Further, the person having the experience feels "sometimes as if he were grasped and held by a superior power."

5. **Life is Seen as Sacred**-The experiences become almost like witnessing a miracle. There is also a realization of the sacredness of life.

6. **You Understand Paradox**-The idea of separation disappears. Things become non-dual. Things become both light/dark, here/absent, human/divine, limited/eternal. This knowledge comes with total certainty.

7. **The Experience Is Indescribable or Ineffable**-The things you witness are beyond the words used to express our ordinary 3D reality. William James told it this way, "The subject of it immediately says that it defies expression, that no adequate report of its contents can be given in words."

8. **Experience Is Temporary**-The mystical experience tends to be transient. Most people end up returning to their habitual way of life. However, the experience leaves them forever changed inside. In his early research, William James discovered, "Mystical states cannot be sustained for long."

9. **The Experience Is Life-Changing**-The majority of people describe it as one of the top five experiences of their life. It is right there with the birth of a child or the death of a parent.

Following are the events that happened, broken down into acts.

Session 1 - Compassion

My first dose of psilocybin brought about much fear about the dreaded "bad trip," often discussed when the psychedelic subject comes up. Generally, we understand that the higher the dose, the more likely some dark moments could appear in the experience. I took about 3 grams, which was more than some of my acquaintances were taking, but it was below the 5-gram dose that Terence McKenna says starts to clear out your mind. The *clearing out* is where the dark moments can show themselves as the person faces the past events and thoughts or beliefs that have been repressed.

As with all future sessions, I considered it to be like going to school. I was not interested in being entertained. It was not done to be a better person, nor to feel good. I was curious about how psilocybin fits into the topic of consciousness and reality. I realized that the only way to figure out what was going on here was to experience it firsthand.

Like school, I had a set time. My trip would start at 8 PM and would end at 1:30 AM. I would then be able to get some sleep once it was over. At precisely 8 pm, I mixed the mushrooms in cherry yogurt and ate it. Then I got into bed and under the covers. I put on a blindfold, my headphones and turned on the *Johns Hopkins Psilocybin Playlist*. This is used in standard research studies when testing psychedelics in the laboratory.

It occurred to me to go into one of the many studies that Johns Hopkins was doing on psilocybin. Still, I did not because:

1) I didn't qualify for any.

2) Being halfway across the country and going there would be very expensive. Therefore, I tried to duplicate what they were doing in my own home.

As soon as I took the mushrooms, I realized a couple of things that I think helped.

- I used the proper *set and setting* to do the session. I had followed the protocol of lying down in bed, using a blindfold, and putting on headphones to listen to music. The use of music to guide one through a trip was developed and used back in the 1950s when researchers worked with LSD. The music I had chosen was the *Johns Hopkins Psilocybin playlist*.

  As the website *Psychedelic Support Education* spells out, "the music is there to evoke and support emotional experiences, including emotionally intense memories, thoughts or experiences." However, it should not be too pushy in what type of emotions it calls forth. Most of the music used in psychedelic-assisted sessions is instrumental, and when there are vocals present, they are in an unfamiliar language. This is to make sure that the music does not convey a specific meaning or tell a specific story. The music should also be culturally appropriate, making it easier to follow and convey emotion rather than drawing attention to itself by use of too "strange or jarring melodies or tones."

- I acknowledged that once I had taken the mushrooms, there was no escape door from what was about to happen. This realization helped me to just "own the experience," whatever that experience would be.

- I knew that what I would experience would be thoughts created by consciousness and that studies in consciousness cannot hurt you. I started to repeat the mantra "trust, let go, and be open." The idea was for me to be curious about what I would be experiencing and that if I kept this concept in mind, everything would be fine. This turned out to be true.

This was the only session that I did not record the audio for. Therefore, I am not sure of the exact details because the psilocybin experiences, like dreams, fade once the left brain comes back online. The EEG pattern goes back into the beta state of being awake and aware, and the memory of what has just occurred goes down the drain like a flushing toilet.

Act 1

The first thing I recall was a pain in my left pectoral muscle. This is not unusual as I have had a left shoulder problem for many years. I was much more aware of the pain in the relaxed state I was in, which made it seem worse. Having never done psilocybin before and realizing that I was home alone, my ego started to fear the possibility that this may be heart-related. I did some deep, slow breathing, and I had no problem, but the pain and the fear lingered. I decided that if this were my time to have a heart attack, then that would happen.

I had been diagnosed with congenital heart failure several years back. Two days of tests were set up in the hospital, and then I was sent back to the cardiologist to hear the results. Would it be confirmed that I had the severe condition he thought that I had?

As I thought of this pectoral pain, my mind seemed to wander back to the memory of the cardiologist's waiting room, where I sat in total fear, waiting for my name to be called. I thought of all the people who sit in waiting rooms just like this and are then given the worst news they can imagine.

Years after this event, I started to use this thought of 'waiting in the waiting room' in compassion meditations. The difference is that in the psilocybin state, the emotions are exposed, almost like someone took the insulation off a live wire. The feelings are much rawer, very similar to reliving the experience on steroids.

When I went into the cardiologist's office, he said the test had come back clean, but he still thought I had something. He told me I was no longer required to make appointments. The relief was so great that I had used it to trigger any thankfulness meditation that I do.

During Session #1, I did not relive the thankfulness part of the experience, just the compassion. Later, I would learn that this was the theme of the first session – compassion. I would have four compassion events in all.

I found myself thrust into an event where I felt the shock and pain of all the people who go into a doctor's office and find out that they are facing the bad news of a life-threatening diagnosis. I could feel their fear and devastation, and was filled with compassion.

It was my first experience of feeling extreme emotion. It was like the insulation around the feeling was now heightened and very raw. This tremendous emotion followed me through all of my psilocybin experiences and seemed to be more enhanced and rawer the higher the dosage.

Act 2

The second compassion event I had was a memory of when I visited the Mexican border in 2018, just south of Tucson. There did not seem to be any connection between it and the doctor's office lesson I just experienced. I was deeply frightened in the cardiologist's waiting room, and the next thing I recall is coming back across the border after spending the day in Mexico.

That day that I crossed into Mexico and returned was an American holiday, and many people were waiting in line to return to the USA. I spent hours in this line until I encountered a border official.

As we got near the front of the line, the tensions were building because most of us in line were well-off westerners who were tired and hot after standing there for so long. Secondly, this was in November, and the temperature was dropping from a hot afternoon to a relatively cool evening. Thirdly, I began to see poor Mexicans entertaining us in line, hoping that people would give them money.

One older, blind lady was playing a small organ and singing. Then, there was a man who was also blind and who did not have arms. He had no instrument but was even singing closer to the border station. I gave both money and was moved, as I had never seen poverty and disability in what appeared to be a society where there was little in the ways of assistance.

As we rounded the final corner where we could see the door into the border station, I noticed that many people were sitting along the wall of the building behind a fence. As we approached, it became apparent they were refugees seeking asylum.

There had been a lot of debate around this time about allowing refugees into the country, mostly Arabs and Latinos. Trump had allegedly called for people to be shot as they crossed the border, and when told that was illegal, proposed a giant moat to be built with alligators. It was a big change from the 1956 Republican platform, which stated, "We believe also that the Congress should consider the extension of the Refugee Relief Act of 1953 in resolving this difficult refugee problem which resulted from world conflict. To all this, we give our wholehearted support."

The President had stated that if people intended to claim asylum, they had to come legally through the border crossing. They should not try and slip into the country unprocessed.

There was one man, two ladies, and two children. One was a girl about 12 years old, and what appeared to be her brother, who was about seven. The girl was playing with her brother bouncing a small ball. She had no right arm and was bouncing the ball with her left. Many stories were being put out in the media that these refugees were a threat to the country, which led me to wonder how a twelve-year-old girl with one arm could be a threat to the mighty United States of America.

I felt great compassion for her and great anger for the situation she appeared to be in. Since we were at the border, there were signs that cameras were not to be used. I was moved by the situation. I took out my camera and took a picture.

The two women talked, and the man was sitting there staring off into space as the long line passed him on the other side of the fence. He looked like his life had just ended. No one in the group appeared to be over 30.

In front of us, the couple from Tucson had been in Mexico to get dental work done. One of them went to the fence and asked the man what country they were from. He replied, "El Salvador," and then went back to staring into space.

My compassion for the situation then was strong, and I remember thinking about how their wait to be processed would be longer than our two hours, which we were complaining about. It is one thing to read about this in the newspaper, but another thing to see with your own eyes. Experience is what changes attitudes and mine was now significantly changed.

When I got back to Tucson a couple of hours later, I could not stop thinking about the family and if they had gotten through the border or not. When I heard that children and adults were being separated, I realized that what I saw was probably the last time this family was together. I feared that this family might now be in four separate cages.

In the psilocybin session, I was back, but this time the insulation of my emotions was gone, and I was back at the border where I could feel the pain of the family. The compassion for them was beyond words. I don't recall anger, just great compassion.

Act 3

The next thing I knew, I was on a ship in the Mediterranean. It was nighttime, and I was behind a woman and two children. I sensed the whole event. I don't think I saw it. This was common to all my experiences; in that, I was sensing things and feeling the emotions of the things I was seeing. It is hard to explain.

I sensed the woman was Arab as she had a headcover on. She was sitting near the front of the ship on a bench near the railing. I felt no other people. It was just me, the woman, and the two children. It was like we were in some bubble away from everything else that was going on.

The woman had her arms around her two children, one on each side. She was holding them tightly. It was nighttime, and we were in a massive storm. The wind and rain were pelting the three people, and I could feel it as well.

I sensed that this was another refugee, fleeing some African country seeking a better life. Again, the compassion wells up. I could do nothing but watch. I kept saying, "I am sorry. I am so sorry you have to go through this."

Suddenly, I was the woman. I could feel what she was going through and the fear that was in her mind. She was thinking, "we are not going to make it." (to the new home she had dreamt of when she boarded the ship).

At that moment, a huge wave came over the side of the ship directly onto her. She thought, "not only will we not make it, but we are also about to die." The wave hit, and the vision ended.

<u>*Act 4*</u>

With the emotions at what felt to be a 10 out of 10, and in a total state of compassion for what I was seeing, I was suddenly in what appeared to be a holding facility where children were being held. Again, I could only sense one child, but I knew there were many other children there as well.

Just like when I saw the woman on the ship, it felt like I was in a bubble or a matrix reality separated from what was going around me.

What I sensed was a boy standing in front of me. It appeared to be the boy I had seen at the border, except now he seemed a bit younger. He had short hair and was just standing there looking up at me. Again, the compassion swept through me, and I started to cry.

The most haunting part of the whole experience is that he did not say anything. He did not say "help me" or "get me out." There was no expression on his face. He was just looking up at me as if he was waiting for me to say something.

I was overwhelmed with sadness and compassion; I did not know what to say. I just looked at the boy, crying, and he looked back with no expression.

Finally, I put my hand on his forehead and said, "I am so sorry. I knew you were there, and I did nothing. I am so sorry."

I am not sure how long this last vision went on, but it kept replaying. The psilocybin was wearing off, and I was in and out of this revolving vision. I wanted the experience to end so

I could do something about it. I took off the blindfold and headset and raced to my computer.

By this time, I had realized that this might have been the boy at the border. I looked for a picture of a boy in one of the cages in which children were being held. I rejected using photographs of multiple kids because that is not what I experienced. Finally, I found a picture of what looked like the boy I had seen.

I posted on my FaceBook page, "I knew you were there, and I did nothing. I am so very sorry." As I posted it, I felt great relief, and it was overwhelming.

The posting caused some controversy as it was a bit cryptic. People came up with all sorts of ideas about what they thought the posting meant, so I contacted my assistant Sinead, and we did an interview two days later to explain what had happened. I posted it on my YouTube site, and everything went quiet. It seemed at that point people either didn't believe it, still thought I was in a dark place after using psilocybin, or went back to UFO sightings and government disclosure.

I went into a psychedelics support group and told the story. There wasn't any significant reaction one way or the other, which made me wonder if I had just had an extended meditation with what I thought was psilocybin. I assumed that I would see colored shapes or animals. I did not see any colors, no animals, and as I mentioned above, I seemed to sense everything as if someone were to say, "imagine a tree in your mind." What I had experienced seemed to be playing off memories and ideas I already had.

I was left very confused. I had never heard any reports of a trip where people had had my type of experience. It made me determined that in the next session, I would up the dosage.

As time went on, I came to recognize that the image of the kids in cages might have been a more potent sign for me to speak out about what was going on with refugees on the southern US border.

I came to this conclusion when I understood that others had experienced similar events where they were prompted to action.

1) A famous researcher I knew told a story in a private support meeting at a UFO conference I attended. He had been blind for 25 years. While on a medical trip to Philadelphia, he suddenly recovered his sight while in a restaurant. After proving to his wife that he could suddenly see, he reported that he could see reptilian creatures sitting at various places in the restaurant in the restaurant where they were attached to the hotel. He looked to the one sitting in a booth beside him, and the reptilian said, "Now you see. Go tell someone." He lost his sight again a few minutes after the event and is still blind today.

2) Rick Strassman, who did the initial research on DMT in the 1990s, talked about an experience (also mentioned in the section of my book, *Contact Modalities: The Keys to the Universe*) where he ran into a being during a DMT experience who said to him, "Now do you see? Now, do you see?" It led him

to begin his DMT research and write the book *DMT: The Spirit Molecule,* both of which are now very well known in the community.

Session 2 - Grief- Despair – Dark Night of the Soul

This was my second attempt at attaining an understanding of what is really going on in this reality through psilocybin. I upped my dose to 4 grams. I didn't go to the 5-gram level as my ego was still raising fear and concern over the situation. As I didn't have much experience, it was easy to listen to my skeptical, doubting mind. I stayed below what was considered by many to be the party-dose or breakthrough dose.

This ego battle would be pretty consistent as I got ready for all of my high-dose sessions. Michael Pollan described the same struggle when he did high-dose sessions for his research. "And the problem with your ego," said Pollan, "is it has command of your rational faculties, so it makes really good arguments that are hard to ignore."5

This time I planned to have the experience on an empty stomach. I decided to begin at 3:00 AM. This turned out to have drawbacks as I had constant pain in my stomach during the experience and throughout the next day. I thought the stomach pain was part of it during the experience but later learned that some people get stomach aches from mushrooms.

The pain added to the darkness of the experience because I was confused by the pain. I mentioned that no one said anything about physical pain during the psilocybin trip on the recording I made.

As the experience started, I again relaxed and felt all the parts of my body. Once again, I felt pain in my left pectoral muscle. It felt much worse than usual, and I also thought of my heart, but I remembered from Session #1 that it didn't mean anything.

The next thing I knew, I was hovering motionless in the rafters of a vast cathedral. Like all the experiences I have had, I could sense where I was and the place's condition but did not see it.

What I sensed was that I was in the back of a massive cathedral about 50 feet below the enormous vaulted ceiling. It was tranquil and dark. I could not see the ceiling but sensed it and its structure. I did not see the floor or walls but knew it was in a vast cathedral. I only perceived it, but it was authentic.

As soon as this happened, I knew that this would be a dark experience. I had read about the *bad trip survey* that Johns Hopkins University had conducted. I thought, "Oh, oh. I have heard about this." I instinctively knew what I was about to experience was going to be related.

I had enough knowledge to know how to handle this. I told myself to own the experience. I was the one that had asked for it. After this, the fear seemed to diminish. I started to repeat the mantra, "Trust, let go, and be open."

I also put this pain into perspective. I thought to myself that at least I wasn't where Dale Hawerchuk was. Hawerchuk had been the captain of the local professional hockey team – The Winnipeg Jets. In 2019, he had been diagnosed with stomach cancer. Reports came out that he had beaten the disease, but a week before my Session #2, the announcement was made that his cancer came back. He died a week later.

I told myself that I would only have pain for five hours and should be lucky with the situation I was facing.

Secondly, I resolved to the fact that the next five hours were going to be tough. Suddenly, I seemed ready to deal with it, and I saw it as a welcome experience.

The second thing I did was to start an audio recording. That seemed to end any fear that was beginning to manifest. On the tape, I would have to restrain myself and not freak out. After talking on the recording for 30 seconds, I realized that I was removing myself from the immediate discomfort by taping and now felt like I was someone watching from the other side of the event.

This is the same technique that hypnotists use to handle challenging memory situations for clients. When the individual experiences a very stressful memory situation, the hypnotist explains that they can watch the event from above it. They are peeking through a curtain, watching what is happening, observing it, and not experiencing it.

I recorded two hours and 45 minutes of the event. All that I remembered from this was that the whole lesson seemed to deal with grief and despair. Other than being up in the rafters of a cathedral, I could not remember any other images.

During the experience, I attempted to get back into compassion. I was puzzled that it was no longer there. I thought of some of the things that had occurred in Session #1 but could not hold onto any compassion. It was like I was on the grief/despair train and nothing else existed. As with my other sessions, my attention was glued to the day's lesson, and my mind wasn't allowed to wander off to other things, which usually is what happens in my daily life and during my meditations. The high doses seem to keep a person glued to the radio station, and there is no mind-wandering allowed.

The critical point that I picked up on this second trip was that I was receiving lessons, which I wanted. This pattern of each trip comprising one particular theme continued.

Session 3 - Death

Death is a central topic in many psilocybin experiences. This mostly occurs when taking higher doses which would also be considered *breakthrough doses*.

People have described being ripped apart by a panther, seeing their body being chopped up, or seeing themselves die and then being forced to watch the body rot. This leads to an ego death, where one learns the lesson that you are not your body and you are One with all that is. You come to realize that the body is just a meat suit that we wear and that Shakespeare was right when he said, "All the world's a stage, and all the men and women are but actors. They have their entrances and exits, and each man plays many roles."

This crushing of the ego is terrifying for people when it occurs, but most would probably still describe the experience as one of the most important lessons in their life.

In Session #3, I moved the dosage back to about 1.5 grams. I had been somewhat shaken by my dark Session # 2 and decided to do a smaller dose before doing the large amount that would hopefully bring the breakthrough experience.

The drawback to the lower dosage is that I was experiencing my mind wandering. I was having a hard time staying at the station. I would suddenly catch myself thinking about other things or wondering how long the session had been going on. I noticed when I was in at one hour and fifty minutes and considering pulling the plug on the session because nothing seemed to be happening. At about two hours and fifteen minutes, the sensing of images started.

I did not experience the ego's death in Sessions #1 or #2 but did get something that resembled it in the lower-dose Session #3. This is another session where I did not record much, so some of what happened may be missing.

Act 1

The death experience came in what appeared to be like six small acts in a play.

The first thing I recalled was lying in a casket. Something may have happened before, but I don't remember, so this was the opening scene. I didn't have to watch myself being ripped apart or watch my body rot. I woke up in a casket, which was kind of like winning the lottery of possible ego deaths – if that is what it was.

As before, I only *perceived* being in the casket. I did not see it. Thinking back, I feel confident that I perceived everything and saw almost nothing.

I perceived being in the casket because I was lying in the open coffin looking up. I did not turn my head, get up and look around, or anything else. I just lay there.

I could not possibly have seen the outside of the coffin or where it was, or anything else. Yet, I was in an open casket.

As I lay there, I got the sense that it was unusual but not frightening. I recall thinking, "I don't feel death. This feels okay. It is kind of relaxing."

Knowing that I was in a casket, I also noticed that I was in a giant cathedral. My head was towards the alter, and my feet were facing the entrance to the church. There was no one in the cathedral. It was tranquil and dark except for the light coming in from behind on the coffin's left side. It was coming in from what I sensed was a large stained-glass window, but I felt the glass was not colored.

The light came in at an angle and ended about 10 feet in front of the casket. I remember being very puzzled that there was no light coming in from the coffin's right as I sensed there was a large window there as well.

In short, the experience was pleasant, relaxing, and yet puzzling.

Act 2

The second scene came just like the first. I was just suddenly there. There didn't appear to be any transition between the two events.

I found myself suddenly in a hospice or a hospital. If I were to guess, it was a hospital. I was on the right side of a bed, and there was a hand sticking out beneath a white sheet. I could not see the person and do not know if it was a man or a woman. Like other experiences, I sensed being in a bubble or matrix where the person and I both were removed from everything around us.

I did sense that this person was in the last moments of life. My job was to hold the person's hand as they died.

Although there were no words spoken, I knew that this person was very frightened at the situation, terrified of death and what would happen next. I took the hand and confronted the person saying that I had studied death and what happens after death my entire life. I told the person that they had nothing to fear. I promised them it would be alright. The person that I could not see was comforted.

Act 3

Suddenly, I was at the bedside of someone else who was dying. It was another bed with another hand sticking out. Once again, I could not see the person. The situation was identical except for the fact that this person was an atheist. We did not speak. I just knew.

I took the hand and went into my spiel about how I had studied death, and there was nothing to fear. Although no words were spoken, I suddenly realized that this person did not want to hear this. They did not care. They simply wanted me to hold their hand and be with them in these final moments of life.

I took the hand and, without words, agreed to simply be there in the moment. It felt good.

Act 4

Next the scene changes, and I was hovering high above the Earth. I thought I was looking from east to west. I could sense that the Earth was alive. I could feel that children were being born and that people were dying in a process that had been going on for billions of years. It was like a machine of life and death.

As I watched, I could see the souls of dead people all over the part of the Earth that I could see rising into outer space. I could see hundreds at one time spread evenly over the surface, rising off the surface. They looked like long wisps of smoke climbing up from the surface of the planet. No one said anything. I just sensed it, but the sense came with absolute certainty.

Like the first three acts, there was no sorrow for what I was seeing. It was almost as if I saw how David Copperfield made a building disappear by watching from behind the stage. Now when he did the trick, I could say with certainty, "oh, that's how he does it."

There appeared to be a life and death process that had no good and bad sides to it, no happiness or sorrow. Death was a vital part of the living Earth. The fact that I felt no sorrow didn't seem to bother me. It was like I was being shown the life and death machine, and it was like an assembly line working on automatic pilot.

Act 5

The next thing that occurred is that I was looking south over the United States. The number of wisps of smoke that I interpreted to be dead souls was happening at a faster rate, and I thought about the Coronavirus, even though the country had many other reasons for death like shootings and veterans committing suicide.

Once again, there was no compassion, sadness, or empathy. The assembly line was just moving faster here. Thinking back, I did not sense the birth aspect at all as I did when I witnessed the whole earth-wide vision in Act 4. I just observed.

Act 6

This was the most dramatic of the death scenes. The vision was noticeably short, but it repeated over and over. I could feel myself coming out of the intense part of the experience and finally took off the blindfold as I was tired of watching this final image over and over.

I found that as the psilocybin is wearing off, it becomes tough to remain tuned to the channel. I guess that as the left brain is coming back online, it becomes harder to stop the ego monkey mind from wandering around thinking of other things. It then requires an effort to tune back into the music and stay with the experience's emotion and visions. Though when in the middle of the experience, it is impossible to think of anything else.

What I perceived was a giant wave or surge that came upon the house. It was nighttime, so it was very dark. The small white house was one-third the size of the surging wave. The surge rises, and the wave's left side comes in from the side and engulfs the house. The house does not break up. It just is suddenly gone into the dark blackened surge of the sea. It is tranquil. The house is gone.

The scene played over and over, and it flashed me back to the Island of Galveston, where I had once departed on a cruise. It was a beautiful place. Just after the cruise, a hurricane was reported to hit Galveston directly. The reports called for everyone to evacuate and that those who refused would die. They were calling for a surge something like eight feet across the island. Many people stayed.

When I was viewing this wave, I felt sad but not shocked or overwhelmed. Like the other visions, this appeared to be part of what always happens in the world. I thought of the people who had not evacuated, and I was viewing their final moments. I will certainly never forget the vision of this wave and the complete silence as the house disappeared without a sound.

Session 4 - Magnificence

I think where the problem area lies, is that people think it lies in taking too much. It lies in taking too little because if you take too little, you can resist it you can struggle with it, and then it can turn into a real mess because you (ego) are afraid of it... the problem is that the ego feels threatened by the boundary dissolution and its ace is your self-identification with it, and it can actually say to you "you are dying and here's the evidence."

-Terence McKenna

Getting Ready

Here is the story of preparing for Session #4. The whole idea behind me using psilocybin was to treat the chemical as a vehicle to break through into the psychonauts' Universe and get answers to how it works. I had used meditation, lucid dream techniques and had tried hypnosis using the Michael Newton method, but none had worked.

People knew that I was using psilocybin, as I had explained some of my experiences on my WHITEHOUSEUFO YouTube channel. A few people knew I had done four sessions in total.

I announced that I would do the "hero dose" made famous in the lectures of psychonaut and philosopher Terence McKenna. That put me in a position where I had to follow through.

I decided to start at 8:00 pm on a Saturday and settled on the date about a week before. That week turned out to be complicated.

The reason it was difficult is that my ego realized that it was about to die. It could be said that there are only two doses of psilocybin. One where you take less than 5 grams, and the ego is still part of the trip influencing what is going on, and the 5-gram dose where the ego is crushed and not allowed to control what is happening. In the breakthrough dose, my ego would be eliminated and not allowed on the stage where it could continue to pretend that it is real and no one off stage is responsible for placing the actors in the play.

The true "I Am" resides in the background, knowing that it put a player on the stage of life, and it sits back and watches the performance. On the other hand, the ego is the actor who wants to play the lead role hoping this reality was real. I have come to believe, against all common sense and logic, that the character the ego has chosen to play is real, but that the idea of reality being a play is nonsense. Alan Watts described the ego as having the ability to "take himself in completely...to become a genuine fake." The ego can play the role so well it comes to believe this is the real world.

The ego is into fear and negativity, so it tried to convince me to delay or cancel the execution. I would get thoughts from it about procrastinating and putting it off until the following Saturday. It encouraged me to get all the details of high-dose trips as possible, hinting that I would undoubtedly have a scary experience. It insinuated that I should do more study on the subject of psilocybin, even though I had studied the issue for years and had written about it in two previous books.

The ego wanted me to specifically study the *Johns Hopkins bad trip survey* so I could learn all the bad things that could happen if I decided to go along with the execution. It reminded me of an old rumor that three people had committed suicide while on psilocybin and that people have had to watch their body rot or be chopped up.

It warned me about the high dose I was planning to do and raised questions about whether or not this would be a "safe dose." What is a safe amount, I thought? Who determines a safe dose? Would it be as safe as all of the pharmaceuticals that kill 130,000 Americans a year?

I realized that this information was given from the left-brain scientists and politicians who had their drugs to promote. As had been done for 50 years, they would recommend that psilocybin was, according to the National Drug Intelligence Center at the Department of Justice, a Schedule I substance under the Controlled Substances Act. Schedule I drugs, including heroin and LSD, have a high potential for abuse and serve no legitimate medical purpose in the United States.

Therefore, their egos would claim that zero was the only safe dosage for psilocybin. I reverted to what Terence McKenna said, "I think where the problem area lies is that people think it lies in taking too much. It lies in taking too little because if you take too little, you can resist it, you can struggle with it, and then it can turn into a real mess."

As the date and time got closer, the anxiety created by my ego was intensifying. I was starting to believe that I might be executing the real me; after all, couldn't the ego serve as a warning?

In the afternoon of the event, I bought new batteries for my tape recorder. This would become significant during the experience. I planned to do it a couple of hours after dinner to avoid the stomach pain, hopefully.

I went for a walk to relax and kill time but was still back 30 minutes early. By then, I could cut the ego-induced stress and evil thoughts with a knife. Rather than wait another 30 minutes, I went to the fridge, pulled out the yogurt, and mixed in the mushrooms. I ate it as fast as I could, thinking, "here we go!" It was a bit tough eating that many mushrooms.

Afterward, I spoke directly to my ego. "There you go," I thought. "What are you going to do now?" After starting the Johns Hopkins playlist, I headed for the bed, turned out the lights, put on my headset, pulled down the blindfold, and pulled the covers over me in the bed. I started repeating the chant in my mind, "Own it. Trust, let go, and be open." The trip had begun.

The Trip

If you know what you are doing, you have been careful about who you are with, the setting is good, the substance is pure, and the preparation has been taken seriously; there is little chance of anything going wrong.
-Neil Goldsmith

Turn off your mind, relax and float downstream. It is not dying. It is not dying. Lay down all thoughts, surrender to the void. It is shining. It is shining.
-John Lennon Lyrics to "Tomorrow Never Knows"

As with all of the previous trips, I don't have much memory of how things started. After reviewing the recording I made of this experience, I was able to fill in the gaps. I did wait for my pectoral muscle to jump in and want some attention, but since going to the chiropractor, that didn't happen.

What did happen is something that I didn't remember until the next day. At first, I thought I had gone directly into a mystical Samadhi state.

The recollection that came to me was that I had had a choking sensation much like before. I thought, "Oh, are they doing that again?" As soon as I discounted this, it quickly disappeared.

Perhaps another attention-getter would work. I started to feel heavy pressure on my chest as if I had some severe lung disease or someone was sitting on my chest. It was uncomfortable. Knowing that this might be another game, I asked myself to breathe to see if I was indeed having trouble. I did and noticed that I could breathe just fine despite the pressure on my chest. (On the recording, I reported not being able to breathe well, but that is not my recollection) I remember wondering, "why would this happen? What was the point?" Maybe it was just my ego striking out for attention, to raise fear, so it could get me to manifest some evil demons or aliens.

While integrating this body discomfort, I realized that people who are doing ayahuasca experience this as well. Many have diarrhea and vomit. This may have been cleansing, but it seemed more like the ego testing whether I would go into fear and anxiety mode, or it may have been fear and anxiety caused by my left brain. I say this because as soon as I said I would either ignore the discomfort or just treat it as background wallpaper for the experience, it stopped.[2]

---

[2] There is another body signal that works the same way. People who do out of body experience or channeled automatic writing will report creating a state where they put the body to sleep while keeping the mind awake. They report that the body will send a signal or roll over on the side (called rollover signal), and that this signal must be ignored to stay awake. Another reported event is that the body will create an itch to test if the body is asleep. If the mind uses the hand to scratch the itch, the body stays

I knew the next thing I started to sense was color, which I had not seen before except for a short while in Session #3, where I saw the light beside the casket. I felt what I referred to as a "xendra smoke" described when ET beings are reportedly manifesting into our 3D world. The edges of the smoke, and the inner folds, had bright fluorescent colors. I was overjoyed.

The After Effects

Unlike Sessions #1, #2, and #3, this session had some aftereffects that are worth noting.

I took Gravol to settle my stomach, so there was no stomach pain as in Session #2. When the trip had ended, many things were different. Something similar was the inability to sleep, and once I did sleep, it was in broken segments of about two-hour chunks. I attributed this to trying to understand what had happened and replay the beautiful parts of the experience that I did remember. I was also starving again.

However, I noticed that as in dreams, once the left brain comes back online, the connection to the images starts to fade out quickly like a dream. These images are compelling and meaningful when you experience them, but they quickly disappear when you wake up.

---

awake. The itch must be ignored; the body will go into sleep paralysis and the mind can travel out of body or enter the lucid dreams state.

The main thing that I noticed was that I was completely drained of energy. The research I have done shows that this may be common in high-dose sessions. This surprised me. I thought that the powerful emotion and meaningful experience would provide energy for me once I returned to 3D. Instead, it seems to have pulled power from me. This went on for days and decreased as a function of time.

This lack of energy was accompanied by a tingling sensation, which I interpreted as the possibility that I was still vibrating higher than my usual 3D self. The differential between the two was confusing, with two separate frequencies operating at the same time.

The worst side-effect was a headache, which went away with an Advil. After several hours, it came back less severe and required another. The stomach pain was absent during the session, but the next morning it returned and lasted over a day. This, I attributed to being my chronic anxiety, which I had hoped the session would solve. It appeared that this did not take place.

The weirdest and most important aspect of the aftereffects of the high-dose session was the mental oddities. I continued to have trouble sleeping with some nights of broken sleep where I would wake up after a couple of hours, and it would be tough to get back to sleep.

This, however, came with a positive effect. Within seconds the "flow state" and "feeling of certainty" were back. Both of these feelings I experienced with my noetic download experiences in 2012 and 2017. When these feelings come, it is time to grab a pen and start writing.

This state is hard to describe to someone who hasn't experienced it. People characterizing the "mystical state" define it as an objective reality where there is a strong feeling that one is experiencing a much more complex and profound truth of our reality.

Later, I discovered that there was a book written by Mihaly Csikszentmihalyi called *Flow*. In this, the psychologist presents investigations of what he refers to as "optimal experience." During these flow states, Mihaly states people typically experience deep enjoyment, creativity, and a total involvement with life.

This flow-state work by Csikszentmihalyi was important to me as I had discovered it by experience through my personal "inspirational" or "in the zone" moments and had given it the same term.

Experiencing this flow state allows an individual to distinguish between experience and belief. There is a powerful feeling that the certainty felt during the flow state is true, objective reality instead of subjective belief. It is as if what is being perceived is the real world.

The psilocybin experiences recreated these feelings for me along with what can only be described as raw emotion. The sessions just made the flow state more fluid and the certainty more certain. The level of the dose seemed to determine how fluid and specific the ideas would be.

On the first night this occurred, I got the impression to write the book. It came like, "these session ideas look like they are setting up a book – how weird." I thought, Should I do a book? I felt the certainty and a positive feeling once I internally resolved to talk to my assistant Desta about it.

I did discuss with Desta, and she asked about the title. I had thought of The Psilocybin School because up to that point, that is what it had been.

In the middle of the next night, maybe 10 seconds after I awoke, as I was headed to the bathroom, the title popped into my head - *Breakthrough: The Psilocybin School*. I had been given the title, and it summed up my entire effort to set up the mushroom sessions.

People do mushrooms for many reasons. For me, there was only one reason and one reason only. Seeing this as a contact modality, I was looking for a breakthrough into a field of knowledge that would help me understand my place in the world.

Two nights later, there was another incident where I awoke to go to the bathroom. Again, I found myself in a flow state of information that appeared to be looking at objective reality, where I saw a lot of Aha! Moments:

- Understanding dreams – In the past, I kept a dream journal to attempt to learn what are called dream signs. Dream signs are weird elements in dreams that a person learns to recognize as things that only happen in dreams. Knowing these signs allows the dreamer to realize they are dreaming when they are in the state. If they can do that, they will become lucid and then do all sorts of exciting things like fly around, change characters in the dream, or ask questions of the Universe.

I stopped writing dreams down because they were so nonsensical, and I could not get lucid as the technique promises.

As I woke to go to the bathroom, I remembered the dream I just had, and knew what it meant. The message was clear, and it was a first for me.

From the Audio Recording

- 0:00- "Strange choking feeling again. Pressure on my chest. Everything is moving in slow motion."
- This is the first time I have seen the colors. "red, green...you sense the colors you don't see them. There is some vibration in the back. Very intense sort of body vibration. Yellow-green. Like long giant snowflakes. A sort of vibration on the chest."
- "No images. There doesn't seem to be a theme to this one."
- "You are sort of able to tune into the music as it becomes more intense. The music seems to affect what you are seeing. It is almost like it is dancing with your thoughts. Still have the sick to my stomach and choking thing going on."

- 3:00- "Let's describe this. It is like a lace (pattern). Psychedelic. Yeah, that's where they get the word from. Very bright. Well, I'll be damned. It has toned right down. Once I mentioned it, it toned right down. The more music gets intense, the more there is a tightening in my chest. The choking is in my chest, not my throat. When I breathe in, I can't breathe in. The music is getting more intense. More and more intense. Yellow, purple. It is getting more intense. It seems to bother me when I talk. I will stop and see if it stops; it is right above me, very bright purple. Somewhat hard to breathe. Better than before."

- 8:00 – "Not sure what the lesson of this is. When I talk, I vibrate. Sort of an intense feeling in my stomach, the more the music gets intense. It is like a tightening in my chest. Trust, let go, be open. When I am not talking, it is not quite as intense; if I am not talking, I can get right into the music. The music is getting very intense, and so is what I am seeing. Extremely intense. Extremely intense. White with red streaks. Beautiful. Thank you, thank you. Beautiful. It's a feeling. It's emotion. It's a feeling. It almost makes you want to cry. I think I'll cry. Ohhh, beautiful."

- 10:00 – "You need the music. The music is doing it. Ohhh beautiful. Absolutely. Thank you. Oh my God. Unbelievable. Red, yellow, blue. It's like a rainbow but colors, but colors you would not see on Earth. Very psychedelic. Very, very bright psychedelic (referring to color, not pattern). You forget you are in the music. The music does it. Beautiful, beautiful colors and very intense. Intense, intense, like raw emotion. Beautiful. There are tears in my eyes. Look up at it. What would you do if you didn't have the music? What would you see? Oh, the music, blue, psychedelic purple, red, orange, right above me, coming down at me. Oh, intense, intense. Oh my God. Wooow. Wooow. So, it's color, emotion, and music. Wow. Wow. It's ineffable. How do you describe it?"

- 14:00- "I'm trying to describe and yet tightness in my chest. The tightness in the chest is coming from a vibration. It is like it is vibrating too much. The vibration just started. I can feel it in both hands. The colors are not quite as intense. Oh, it is the music that has dropped down. The music is still going. You have to do this with music. That's half of the experience. That's half the experience. Very weird, there is a soprano singing. Italian. Very, very slowly. Your whole body vibrates. Oh my God. Sinead would miss this because she can't hear. She is singing very high. It's too bad you can't hear her singing. Oh, it just vibrates the entire body. Oh, I see. Sensitive people can pick up the vibration of her voice. Does it have a color? Let's see yellow, purple, green, orange, then purple again. There is real tightness in the chest. Oh, my goodness. Oh, that's why they use this music! Oh, you have an appreciation for the music. It is like you are soaring. It is like you have risen into the sky. It's all different. The colors are gone now. I am up high in the sky with music. It is very, very intense. There is pressure on the chest. Wow. Ah, beautiful music. It is like it is part of the experience. It is like they wrote it for the experience. It seems like they wrote the music for the experience. Wow. There is a very, very intense tightness in the chest. Oh, wow."

- 20:00 – "I see what they are doing! The music is combined. It is like a vibration. Red-green. You don't notice the colors unless you concentrate on them. The key thing is the intense pressure on the chest. Extreme. Extreme. Extreme pressure. It is so different from the first three experiences. On the chest, it is crushing. Crushing. Bight green. Dark. Crushing. Holy sh*t. The weirdest part is that you forget that you are being recorded. You are in the experience. Very, very intense pressure. Almost to the point that you can't breathe. I'm coming down. Is there any sort of message? There is some color coming in from above on the right. (Yawn) Man, you forget where you are."

- "Let me describe where I think that I am and what is going on. Okay, go. I have to wait for the music to pick up. When the music is down, there is not so much of an effect. There is pressure on the chest. There is very intense pressure, so it is not just a visual thing. I don't love this kind of music. Okay. Okay. It's like I am dead, but I'm not dead. Weird. Okay. I don't remember the music being like this. The music is gone completely, almost like I am dead. Ok (speaking VERY slow). I can hear the note going soooo sloooww. Weird. Weird, (whispering) weird. Weird. The music is going so slow like I am dying. I feel like I am dying. I feel like I am dying. Okay. Okay. (whispering) The music is stopping. The music is vibrating. The music can't be like this. This has to be the experience. How would they know? How would they know? It is you are part of the music. You are part of it. It is so quiet. There is no music. Good thing I've got this thing taped; this is so damn weird."

- 29:00 – (A commercial comes on between the music) "Wow. Wow. It is so unique compared to what the first couple of sessions were—using a higher dosage. There he goes. This is angelic music. Colorful. Light. I can still feel the pressure in my chest. Ah. It is just so wonderful. There is a choir with deep base tenors singing. There are sopranos, and they light it up when they sing. There is light with them. Their color is yellow fluorescent yellow. Very, very bright. It's weird. To think that people are listening to this. Ah, that is angelic singing. That is like yellow and green. Ahh. I am so thankful. You suddenly think about it, and you are lying in your bed. And you are. You do forget who you are. You have to think about it."

- (There is a lot of half-sentence in the next section as it is tough to finish a sentence without great concentration. The talking is very slow here as I am

69

transfixed on the music and emotion of the experience) "I am trying to describe this, but it is difficult for those who are listening. I wish people could listen. You don't hear the choir. You don't hear the sound. I can feel the tightness in my chest. Ok. Ah, so beautiful. You completely forget who you are and what you are doing. Trust, let go. Ohhh, I can feel the tightness in my chest. Ahh. So beautiful. I am so sorry you could not hear the music. Ok. It is so weird. Weird. You lose your identity. It is very, very bright. The thing is that you can feel. You can feel the pressure like someone is sitting on your chest. It's hard to breathe. Oh, thank you, beautiful. They are playing music. It would not be the same experience without the music. It is like the vibration of the music (loses thought). It is like the thing lights up. It is weird. Weird. It's like (loses thought). I never thought I would *see* the music. It is not that you see the music. There is this very angelic. It was so weird. You forget. So sorry you cannot hear the music. The more you take (mushrooms), the more the intensity. I see. It is like colors and vibrations. Beautiful. Thank you. The music. Here comes the crescendo as the music intensifies the effect that you have from the psilocybin. It is like raw emotion. This would be color and the emotion that goes with it."

- "It's purple. There is tightness in the chest. Purple. So bloody weird. So weird. So weird. Wow. Wow, thank you, thank you, thank you. God, that was beautiful.

Without the music, you just sort of vibrate. Without the music, you vibrate, but when you put the music together. You need the music. Holy sh*t. You forget who you are. You lose your ego. You become One. There has only been one commercial, but this is absolutely beyond words. It's like a deep tenor choir in a huge cathedral. It not that you see it, but when you want to describe what the sound is, it seems to take that, and there is a deep intense pressure on my chest, almost like I cannot breathe. It is soo weird. It is beyond words. I forget that I am taping this. Wow, I wish to describe it; it is like church music, but when you experience the same music. I am glad I taped this. It is ineffable. It is hard to describe the beautiful angelic soprano choir. You can feel the vibration of your whole body. My entire body is vibrating. You become the music. Desta and I talked about this. You become the music. You forget that you are taping it or who you are. You manifest what you see as unbelievable. This music vibrates your entire body; you have to hear the music, what a different experience. You have to do it with the music. You lose the sense of time. There has only been one commercial. I am trying to describe this, but the sad thing is you cannot describe this without hearing the music. IT is like a paranormal experience because there has only been one commercial...."

- 53:00 – (A commercial comes on) "Even the commercial is cool."

At this point, after going to the bathroom, I somehow didn't turn the audio recorder back on and missed the crucial part of the experience that seemed like a full-blown Samadhi or mystical experience.

As I was coming out during the last hour, I tried to explain what had occurred. Some of the impressions I made from what I remembered were:

- "What you focus on comes into reality. It manifests. It becomes more real. "If you don't think about it, it becomes like a dream."

- "I am in a complete flow state. Things are coming with absolute certainty. When I went to the bathroom, I focused on the real world, but I became dizzy; everything in the universe is vibration and emotion; you have to be here to feel it..."

- "Here is this song. They have played it four times. It is in my upcoming Portal to Ascension music presentation. That's kind of weird."

- "It was all emotion. It was all feeling."

- "When you come out of the psilocybin experience, you start to lose focus. You lose the radio station. You realize you are not the music anymore. You are now just listening to music."

- 'The silence has a vibration. It is bizarre."

- "I feel the energy draining away. I feel that now."

Session 5 - Let Go

Opening note *– In this session, I appeared to be dealing with something that had great intelligence. It was skillfully directing the lesson and had control of my physical body. I do not know what intelligence is, so I call it "the intelligence behind the psilocybin." It could be God, the Universe, my higher self, or an intelligence group. During the session on tape, I usually referred to the intelligence as "you guys." That is how it felt. Whatever the intelligence is, it is highly clever and knowledgeable. That was the most understandable description I could make.*

Of the many books I have written, this is the most challenging chapter I will ever have to put to paper. In a moment, you will know why. Many times, during this 5th session, I would say, "You have to be kidding. You want me to put this in my book? You have to be kidding." The intelligence was not kidding. It was deadly serious.

Once again, I was not looking for better health, a circus-like experience, or to feel good. I was going to school and entered it, waiting for whatever the intelligence behind the mushrooms was prepared to teach me. I was waiting for a lesson. On this night, the intelligence did not let me down.

I was somewhat curious about what would happen in the Session #5 experience. This is because in Session #4, I had experienced a full-blown mystical experience that would rate as the top experience in my life. I was, therefore, very intrigued at how the intelligence would top that event.

My intention started with a line from Jesus. "Not my will, but thine, be done." This was to set the goal that the intelligence would lead, and I would follow. At least, that is what I thought. The ego, which runs the physical consciousness show, had different ideas.

The second intention I had is one I use every time. I repeat the words given to people in the Johns Hopkins research lab when they do a high-dose session. "Trust, Let Go, and Be Open." It is these words that the intelligence would use to crush the ego. I would come to learn that it is easier said than done when repeating mantras.

Finally, I reminded myself that nothing inside consciousness can harm me and that I must always "own the experience." The owning it part is essential because anything can happen in a high-dose session, and the worse reaction is to become a victim. The idea is to accept responsibility for the situation, reducing or eliminating the fear reaction.

Looking back at what happened over my past four sessions, it appeared that the intelligence was giving me lessons as chapters of a book, so this experience, and its lesson, would be Chapter Five.

I had been micro-dosing for a month and became very excited when I determined that I would again do a high-dose session.

I was not aware that the intelligence has a sense of humor, almost like the experiences by tricksters who haunt the paranormal world. I didn't know till later on, but on this night, the intelligence seemed to be saying, "Let's spice up the book. Maybe you can get it on the NYT bestseller list. Do you want a lesson chapter? Watch this!"

Chapter 5 was the result. During the experience, twice I applauded the intelligence openly and laughed as I had never laughed before. It produced a story lesson that Shakespeare couldn't deliver on his best day.

I gathered up what appeared to be three grams of mushrooms but was not sure there was enough, so I took a pill of 250 mg of psilocybin to add to the mix. I took the pill 30 minutes before, and then the mushrooms mixed in cherry yogurt. As I ate the mushrooms, it occurred to me that I didn't particularly appreciate eating them. They seemed to make me want to gag.

I set up the *Johns Hopkins music playlist* but figured that the computer was only playing one song and then stopping. I had them on my audio recorder, but I could not listen to the songs and record the session simultaneously. I ended up wasting a few minutes getting a *Johns Hopkins playlist* off of YouTube and resigned myself to commercials.

Then, I laid down on the bed with the covers over me and put on the blindfold and headset. Unlike the past sessions, the effects came on very quickly. This was probably due to taking the pill early.

As I described on the audio recording, within minutes, I felt that I was floating, and then a few minutes later, I sensed the mist with the edges of fluorescent color. Indeed, I would break into the field in a couple of minutes and learn what the lesson was.

As with other experiences, I was sensing rather than seeing. There was a black background and then some black pattern in the background that I could sense because it was different black shades. The slight color effects were appearing and disappearing into the swirling design.

Suddenly, I had to go to the bathroom. Now would be a good time to go as I was not entirely into the field yet. Going to the toilet is difficult once the plant medicine kicks in because I must shut off the tape recorder and then remember to turn it back on when I get back. I also have to take off the blindfold and headset and turn off the music. When this happens, I am thrown back into the physical world, and it is like being thrown in a pool of icy water.

I quickly headed to the bathroom, and with the light on, I could see brilliant yellow color and a geometric pattern embedded in the color. It is very disorienting but not scary. As this is happening, I no longer feel the need to use the bathroom. The sensation was gone.

So, I head back to the bedroom and, in the dark, turn on the music again, find the tape recorder and start it, put on the blindfold and headset, and get back under the covers. I get drawn into the field and am totally at peace, except I HAVE TO GO TO THE BATHROOM AGAIN, REALLY BAD.

Now I am getting frustrated. I go through the whole shutdown process again and race to the bathroom before being fully in the field. Back in the bathroom, the colors and patterns are pulsing away, and the urge to go is gone again. I struggle to go realizing that I am getting deeper and deeper into the field. Nothing happens.

Back into the bedroom, I go and set up everything in the dark. This time I can't find the headset, and a sense of frustration sets in. What makes it worse is that I'm almost totally disoriented. It is hard to remember who I am or what a tape recorder even is.

Back under the covers again, and I drift back into the comfortable world of the mushrooms. In seconds I have to go to the bathroom again. Now I am beyond frustrated. I realize I have to go as I have maybe five hours left. This is my last chance. The urge to go is powerful, and I wonder if I will even make it.

I go back through the shutdown procedure and the incredible feeling of being back in the physical world. Getting to the bathroom is much more difficult this time, and I realized my first lesson. I am beginning to feel like what is happening right now is happening for a reason.

Act 1

Later in this book, I have suggested protocols on the procedures I follow. It is mostly based on the research protocols used by Johns Hopkins, NYU, and other labs. The only thing I change is not using a person as a guide. I use the protocol encouraged by Terence McKenna, using the high dose alone in a dark room. And if things go south, I remind myself to own the experience.

Most protocols suggest using a friend as a personal guide, and I listened to many interviews by people trying to figure out why they thought it was necessary. One of the talks was from James Fadiman, who said a guide might be wise to help a person find the bathroom. Find the bathroom? Really? Now on my third trip to the bathroom, I could see the intelligence gave me the lesson of why this might help.

I congratulated the intelligence, thinking, "Yah. This is very funny. I get the point." I opened my mouth criticizing the bathroom comment, and now this is my payback.

Back in the bathroom, I could not go even though the sensation was still there. The light and patterns were annoying, like being woken up early when all you want to do is stay in bed and sleep. I had to go back, as I was becoming more disoriented, and everything in the physical world was annoying because of the heightened emotion and sensory state I was in. The situation was now a bit out of control and did not seem resolvable.

Back in the bedroom, I went through the whole setup thing again, struggling even to recall what elements of the setup I had to perform. Back in bed and back into the field, I once again had to go to the bathroom badly. I was running out of time; I could not make many more trips to the bathroom.

Instead of going to the bathroom this time, I got a big towel and pushed it under my underwear, creating a giant diaper. I thought, Now I can relax and stay in bed. The rational, analytical, left-brain ego had figured out a solution to remain in control.

Act 2

It was in realizing that this bathroom nonsense was all being recorded that I knew my ego was under attack. The intelligence was killing the ego, and everyone who heard the tape would laugh at my expense. It was amusing but not funny at all.

Back in the bed, the bathroom sensation returned. Just as the panic got out of control, the main lesson for the night came in. I sensed the words, "Let go!!"

My first reaction was, "Not a chance!" My ego was horrified at the thought.

The sensation came again, "Let go."

I (ego) thought, "you can't be serious."

Again, "Let go." This "Let go" with a "No" reply went back and forth many times.

Every time it happened, the ego got more and more crushed. I (ego) thought, "I am too cool to do that."

Again, I felt an intense feeling to go along with, "Let go. Trust, Let go and Be open."

I was starting to laugh, but the ego stood its ground. I thought, "I can't do that."

Again, "Let go."

My mantra was confronting me. The message was simple – if you trust the universe, you will let go and be open – now trust and let go.

This is a back-and-forth battle that went on for hours, so here is the short version. The ego was being crushed in a taped performance, and it started to rationalize. "I (ego) went to the bathroom numerous times. I did not drink much. How bad could it be?"

The lesson was clear. <u>Kill the ego and let go.</u> The intelligence was clear, in some ways cruel, and it was not backing off.

The sensation to urinate continued unabated, "Let go !!"

Eventually, after searching and realizing there was no escape, the ego said, "OK, I'll let go." It figured this was just a game in the lesson, and nothing would happen.

I thought, "Ok, I am letting go." Nothing happened.

I got a message, "You didn't let go. You didn't try." This was right.

I thought, "I will try again." The lesson was like the sensation when one has to go to the bathroom and barely makes it. When you arrive at the toilet, you stop holding it and let go. The feeling is incredible. You make it to the bathroom just in time. All is well in the world.

I knew that physical "let go" feeling. I repeated that I would do it. I felt the intense bathroom feeling and let go. Nothing happened, and the feeling was still there. I could not let go.

Again, I sensed a message, "Let go!!"

The intelligence was relentless, and it was using the music to intensify the lesson. Right or wrong, I came to believe that intelligence controlled not just my body but the music. There were no commercials again, and the music was exactly what the experience called for.

The prime example was that I was stalling about letting go. A song would come on with a female opera singer or an orchestra that builds up the song to an intense crescendo. I would think there is no way this is a chance. The bigger the buildup in the music, the worse the bathroom feeling became. It would build, build, build, and holding back got harder and harder. It was like some intelligence waterboarding me with music to "Let go," hand over state secrets, and wet the bed.

Many years back, Alan Watts talked about hanging up the phone once you get the message:

> *If you get the message, hang up the phone. For psychedelic drugs are simply instruments, like microscopes, telescopes, and telephones. The biologist does not sit with an eye permanently glued to the microscope; he goes away and works on what he has seen.*[6]

One thing must be added to this wisdom. You can only hang up the phone if they let you. On this night, they would not hang up the phone and kept repeating it, hammering in my mind, which was in a high emotion state, where you cannot turn away. The left-brain voice cannot talk or lead you off to think about other things. The scene that one watches is locked in, and you cannot turn away.

Therefore, once I got the message and the humor of the "let-go" message, I said, "Ok, I've got it, now stop." I did not quite have it, and they just kept going. Unfortunately, the intelligence refused to hang up the phone.

I am not sure in the end if I did let go. Perhaps I did. Nothing happened as I had predicted. The problem was that the prediction was just a guess, and I knew it. I was not 100% sure, and that made me hold back.

This same experience happened to my interview partner Sinead Whelehan, who had been involved in an ayahuasca session in Peru. During the events, she was suddenly looking at some beings. This is how she described the event and how she too could not let go to join the beings:

> *There's a line of beings who are all not bodies at all; they're just light. They're just multi-colored light, but they're not in body shapes. They're in their flowers and fireworks and lines, and squiggles, and twirls, and just shapes. They're moving and moving and moving a lot, and I knew that they were conscious beings because they were talking to me, they were telepathically, and it was this just a huge wave of joy and enthusiasm. It was a very enthusiastic welcome like, 'We're so glad you're here!'*

That's what it felt like. You're finally here. I know that's common among experiencers, that:

When they first meet a being, the beings say, "finally, you made it! What took you so long?" It's sort of that feeling, and you know, "we're so glad you're here," and there is just so much joy, and so much enthusiasm, and such a warm and enthusiastic welcome. So, they repeatedly repeated those phrases, so I was feeling very welcome like I was a hero returning from, you know, another country or something. It was really, really enthusiastic and just immediately a feeling of connection and just welcome - just welcome. So, then that became okay with the same feeling of great enthusiasm it became this urgency. "Okay, we gotta go. You're coming. We're leaving now, and you're coming. Now let's go come on, let's go, let's go, let's go, let's go, let's go. You know we're gonna take you, and we're gonna show you stuff."

So, then what happened when I started getting really distracted by what was happening to my physical body because ayahuasca is hard on your body, and it's a purification thing. So my stomach was going crazy, and I felt like I was sort of being pulled between this plane that I was on with them and all this communication I'm having with them. Them telling me we got to go now and being aware that my physical body was in the Mallorca, sitting on the floor. My stomach is going crazy, and it's really uncomfortable, and they're also saying to me your body has to be clean before you come with us. Your body has to be clean. I said okay, and then I realized that meant that I had to basically let go physically, and I felt then I found all this ego stuff about being embarrassed. You know, not wanting to do that in front of everybody, and then, you know what would happen after that. Well, my mind goes off somewhere else. My body's gonna be here sitting in this light; how's that gonna happen?

*I don't want to do that, so I just suddenly got really self-conscious and, and it is a a little bit stressful because I really, I really wanted to go with them. I thought I have to grab this opportunity, and it, it just feels so good, and they're gonna show me stuff like, who doesn't want to do that? I want to go to space right, but at the same time, feeling very pulled down by to **earth by what was happening with my body and it was, really, um kind of too much, and meanwhile they're like, 'We gotta go, come on, we gotta go, let's go! Come on!'***

So, um I just couldn't do it and so I said to them, 'I'm really, really sorry I can't, I just can't do this; this is too much.' I'm also experiencing all this, you know, the sensory overload, like it was very very, very intense, and I'm breathing, and I'm talking myself through and I wasn't scared, you know, it wasn't like that, it was just very intense and so, I ended up apologizing to them and saying 'I'm really sorry, but I can't do this.'

The tape will tell more of the story. Right now, let me end by explaining the appreciation I had for the message and the powerful way it was delivered. "Touché," I said to the intelligence. One of the biggest life lessons was delivered – kill the ego, trust the intelligence behind the universe, and let go.

To truly let go takes much more than speaking the words.

Act 3

Like previous sessions, I had the slight feeling of choking and the sensation of someone sitting on my chest, which gave the sense of not being able to breathe. Like previous sessions, I carefully looked at my breath and focused on it. Nothing was wrong.

The intelligence had crushed my ego with the *let go and wet-the-bed* game. Now it was time to kill the ego with the experience of physical death, which many in high dose sessions will report. This experience of death was much more comfortable than wetting the bed. I actually enjoyed it.

It came on with increased intense pressure on the chest. It had appeared early in the session but then went away when I focused on taking a breath. An interesting related note is that the breath felt like a thing. I could feel it going into the lungs, and it seemed to have a structure and substance I had never experienced before. I marveled at it while trying to study and describe it into the tape.

Now the pressure on my chest was back, but it was much heavier than before. I had picked up the message of the death of the mental ego and realized that this might be a demo of the death of the body, which I already experienced in Session three, being in a coffin in a cathedral.

It was exciting, knowing that the tape recorder was running[3] , and I could now describe the death of the body. I would die but come back, so there was absolutely no fear.

As the pressure increased, I described the feeling of dying. The struggle to breathe was more challenging, even though I had no trouble talking. The breaths became more complicated and shorter as the pressure increased, and I seemed to lose physical sensations.

Act 4

The fourth lesson was a new one for me. During the numerous times I went to the bathroom, I realized that when you are heavily at the peak of the experience and then come out into the physical world, it is very disorienting.

On a couple of occasions, it wasn't easy starting the music again and finding the headset. At one point, I lost the tape recorder, and because it is hard to focus and put things in order, I just gave up on it.

Luckily, I found it later and started it up just as the music ended. Twice the computer had shut off because there was no action. The screen (which is almost totally unreadable under the influence) would put up a message saying. "Are you still there? Continue playing?"

---

[3] I hoped the tape recorder was running. It is almost impossible to break out of the experience to look at the recording light, this would throw me back into the physical world.

The first time this happened, I struggled to find the OK button and click on it. I was so heavily focused on the experience the second time that I could not be bothered. Now for the first time, I was tripping without music.

The silence was deafening. I realized that silence is not anything. It appeared to have a color (white) and a composition that I could recognize if I met silence on the street. I listened carefully and could not hear my breath. "How weird," I thought. When I became very still and focused (focus is a big thing in this state), I could sense a small high-frequency vibration.

While in the silence, a loud sound alarmed me, which was alarming as it shattered the silence. This was elevated by my heightened emotional and sensory state. When the recorder's button turned back on, it sounded like an alarm clock going off.

I can already make my whole body vibrate in the physical world, so I tried to make my body's vibration more intense. In short, I could. The world of silence is genuine and very weird.

Late in the session, as the plant medicine was wearing off, I broke out of my comfortable bubble to turn the music on again. I went back under the blindfold but realized I had broken the field and could not get the music to pull me back. I was no longer the music but was now listening to music. The flow state was gone, and the sense of certainty about things I was thinking about was gone.

I ended the session to email some friends and warn them that the session was over and that compelling things had occurred.

Act 5

I was not aware of time, but it must have been near the end of the fourth hour when I started to play with the plastic, flow-state within the field. I also became more confident about where I was so I could control some elements of what was going on.

During a download or noetic experience, a feeling comes with the information that a person is receiving. The information that is being perceived is flowing in and comes with absolute certainty.

My awareness was moving around and whatever I concentrated on came into focus. Without that concentration, the attention just flips to one thing after another, continually losing the train of thought.

I tried several things like telepathy and leaving my body but could not concentrate hard enough. My mind just forgot about doing the task after five seconds and wandered on to something else.

In future sessions, I will try and work on this bizarre flow state. The other thing I will work on is describing the "me versus Grant," something that I have noticed many times. Most of the time, it feels like I have the experience, but from time to time, I will be looking and think, there is Grant over there doing something that is happening to him.

Some might explain this as the big Grant and the little Grant. This goes back to the idea that the real person is the observer, and the physical person is the person on the stage. From this comes the great goal of life, which is to remember who you really are.

The final thing to point out in this 5th session is the physical effect. Four hours into the trip, I had a headache and a terrible pain in my upper back. This came from the fact that I was agitated during this whole "Let go!!" drama with the back-and-forth. I don't usually move much during a session (except to applaud the lesson instructor when I finally get it), and I must have been in a weird position that was held for a long time.

There were two hours and forty-five minutes of recorded audio. I describe each moment as the play-by-play of a hockey game that I was experiencing. It provides many more details of what happened than the few bits and pieces that I remember once the medicine wears off. A session's memories are more like dreams that fade quickly once the left brain comes back online.

Aftereffects

The only real notable change that occurred in my daily life from this experience was my dream state. My dreams had changed.

Previously, I had recorded my dreams to search for dream signs to try lucid dreaming.[4] There was a point where I could recall parts of 6-7 dreams a night. Even though I could recognize some dream signs, like my dead father being in a dream, I could not use these to then become lucid in the dream. The dreams appeared to be nonsensical. They seemed irrational, so I stopped detailing them.

The dreams I began to have after Session #5, however, were more positive. They seemed to make more sense or gave me direct lessons or understandings. They were, however, clearly different.

A couple of weeks after Session #5, my dreams had changed. I am not sure if the realization came during the dream or just after awakening, but I thought it was true and that my dreams had changed.

They were brighter, more like daylight compared to nighttime. They made more sense and were more positive. I remember thinking how weird it all was and wondered how this could happen.

---

[4] The idea of dreams signs is that once you learn to recognize them you can understand that you are dreaming during a dream, that they do not make sense, and therefore understand that a dream is occurring. Once the recognition is made, the person can recognize they are in a dream and become lucid. In a lucid, plastic state, a person can then ask questions and control the dream state.

Session 6 – Vibration – The Musical Ecstasy

This may sound like a clickbait title, but I could not find any other term to describe what was going on while in the state. As with other chapters, I wait for "them" (whoever that might be) to tell me what the lesson is, and this appears to be what they wanted for Chapter 6.

I document this immediately after my session because the details disappear like a dream, and I am left only with the feeling. Luckily, there are audio recordings that I make, though I never listen to any of them.

This loss of memory leads to weird situations like the fact that Chapter 4, "Magnificence," was the most awe-inspiring moment of my life, and yet, I do not remember most of the details of that session. This 6th session was more dramatic than the 4th, and the details are fading quickly.

In Session #6, I started with a 15-minute meditation once taking the medicine. I used my Muse headband, which registers how calm my mind is. It was certain that I would be nervous, and my number would not be good. The opposite happened. The Muse recorded 145 birds (indicating a quiet mind) in 15 minutes, about as good as ever, and it showed no mind-wandering breaks.

As with all my previous sessions, there was just one theme, one lesson. I experienced the edging colors in the dark as the trip began. There was nothing else. I still wonder if others who use psilocybin also have only one *theme* per session, or do I get one theme because that is my intention?

It appeared to me after my first three sessions that I was being given lessons that could be set up like chapters of a book. Now I am in Session 6, and once again, I got a lesson that is called *vibration – the musical orgasm.* It was taught to me in numerous states of ecstasy using music.

I wonder if a theme is with every session, and I am always curious about the next lesson. I keep thinking they may eventually run out of lessons and could start repeating them. "They" did not let me down, although it was well over an hour before the lesson began.

I was in a state of heavenly bliss for three hours. As it was happening, I thought back to the Magnificence lesson in Session #4 to compare. During that session, I was feeling a sense of Samadhi or a deep mystical state. This was just as intense, or maybe more, but the only word that seemed to fit was *bliss.*

As with all things in the high-dose psilocybin world, things are ineffable. This is one of the key elements that describe a mystical state. A person struggles to find words to explain what they experienced clearly. The English definition of bliss is "a state of extreme happiness, blissfulness, cloud nine, seventh heaven, and walking on air." That is close, but the Hindi version is even closer to what I repeatedly experienced for three hours:

> *All that is left of the personal soul is a hymn of peace and freedom and bliss vibrating somewhere in the Eternal.*

The keyword that could even begin to explain what I experienced is where the word *orgasm* comes in. There was a repeated pattern where the vibration would build, and then there would be a rush that would move up through my body and continue to intensify the more I concentrated on it.

That vibrating energy maybe my *kundalini*, a Sanskrit word that describes the latent, female, cosmic energy believed to lie coiled at the base of the spine, which, when uncoiled, moves up the spine. It was not.

This energy was accumulating in a field that, at first, seemed to be inside my body and an area around my body. But later, after repeatedly triggering this energy release, I realized that THERE IS A FIELD WHERE VIBRATING ENERGY CAN BE CREATED, USING THINGS LIKE MUSIC. MY BODY FIELD IS INDEPENDENT OF THIS BUT AT THE SAME TIME IS PART OF THE FIELD. There was separation but no separation.

For three hours, I was in this bliss state where I recorded myself describing how to increase the intensity five or 10x as much by "leaning into the vibration of the music or singer," and finally how music causes such ecstasy in the psilocybin state.

There was a slight delay in doing Chapter Six. Firstly, I was planning to increase the dosage to 7 grams, and then I started reading some literature on high doses, which again triggered my ego mind to get scared and talk me out of it. I still might have gone along with it, but I was having stomach trouble all day, and it seemed like a sign to not proceed with this. I have had stomach problems in the past and was starting with a bad stomach.

The session got delayed repeatedly, and I was feeling down that my ego seemed to be winning. I felt a strong desire to get back into another trip.

Usually, I do not do sessions during the week as I often wake up early, but the session kept getting delayed, so I decided to do 2 grams. I figured they could give me a chapter with two grams because the death chapter had come with just 1.5 grams.

I started by adding four microdose pills of 0.5 grams each, and by the time it kicked off, it must have been close to 4 grams. Adding more of these 'boosters5' during the session was because I knew I had a ticket to heaven and thought it only right to try and stay for a while.

Maybe other people report experiencing these states of bliss. If they are, they need to get off their backsides and talk more about it. I have searched yet not found much. Here is my perception of how the system works. These are my impressions of things that were shown to me. This whole

---

5 A booster dose is used when it appears the dosage may not have been sufficient or to extend the time of the trip. My usual booster is 0.5 grams.

chapter is about music and is significant because I do not listen to it, even after writing a book about it. Music is not a factor in my life, but it dominated this entire psilocybin session.

- Based on what I experienced, it appeared to me that there is a field that we are all in.

- When the music is playing, it creates vibrations in the field, and because my body field is in the big area, the music was causing my entire field to vibrate. At first, I thought each note was like a string, but later I concluded that my entire 3D field (that extends outside my body) was vibrating.

- My sense of this field was that it was larger than my body but had no defined edges.

- The field vibrated by the note, not the song. When deep in this state, it was clear that I was listening to the vibration being created by the various instruments and not the music. This was verified to me when in one of the classical pieces, there are just piano notes being played by one hand. The notes were being played slowly, maybe one per second. With each note, my entire field vibrated.

- Because I was listening to the music's vibrations in the field, I had no idea of what the music was. It was just a set of vibrations. It was music that I would probably not listen to in my everyday 3D life. This is significant because most people would want to hear music they like and know, but there would be a risk of engaging the left brain and making you want to sing along, especially if there are lyrics, as words are a left-brain function.

- Instead of hearing the music, I was picking up on the various instruments and voices and their vibrations in the field. The most noticeable tone to create this feeling of lift and bliss was that of soprano opera singers. I usually had to stop talking to my audio recording when the singer hit the high notes, as it was impossible not to be drawn in. Next were choirs, mostly if they were large. Violins have a distinctive pitch that creates an uplifting bliss. Tubas have a tone that vibrates the field with their low tone.

- As noticed in an earlier session, I could sense the composer's mood and emotion as he was creating the piece. Each musical piece was almost like a fingerprint of that moment of his life. These would not be noticeable in the 3D world. In that world, at least to me, it is just music.

- This vibration even applied to the commercials on Spotify (where I listen to the playlist). Even they vibrated, but it had a different feel to the music in the playlist. Then I realized that commercial voices had a vibration as well, and this vibration applied to my voice when I concentrated on it.

- Each note created vibration. Once the note vibrates the field, my field would vibrate as well.

- Then came a critical discovery. I noticed that once my field would vibrate, it would continue to vibrate. A second note would be played, and it would create a second vibration in my field. There would be another note and another. The vibration and ecstasy would grow. A situation would be made where there were 100 different vibrations all going simultaneously in my field.

- Another aspect that would drive up the delight would be male or female choirs that would create heavenly ecstasy. What I was experiencing at the high points was a heavenly place. I noticed that it was not one vibration but multiple vibrations from each of the voices; therefore, 50 people in the choir were 50x more intense than just one voice.

- Another blissful point would be the voices of tenors and particularly the sopranos hitting high notes in crescendos during the classical pieces. The vibration and ecstasy at that point would be so intense I would have to stop talking. It was overwhelming.

- Then, I would be drawn into the music, almost like being swept up into the funnel of a tornado. The direction was up, and the term "swept up in the music" comes to mind.

- Once a song would end, there would be a clear and absolute silence. In that silence, my field was still vibrating from the music. It stood out and was very noticeable.

- An important discovery was repeated many times in Session #6. When I stopped talking and focused on the music, I would be drawn into the music like a vacuum cleaner picking up dirt, and the intensity of the ecstasy would increase five or 10x. How much it intensified was directly related to how hard I concentrated. What I was doing was "leaning into the music."

- The technique of concentration would be akin to asking the reader to thread a needle. When given this task, the reader will hold their breath and concentrate while they complete the chore. Leaning into the music involved holding my breath and focusing as hard as possible on the music vibration. This would multiply the vibration and create an intense vibratory state similar to the building of an orgasm. I would feel myself lifting as my field increased in vibration. The harder I focused, the faster I would go up, and the more the feeling of bliss. I did it over and over and described what I was doing each time on the recording. At the end of the whole session, I had a sore back, which probably came from holding my breath and concentrating so hard.

- One of the most revealing vibrations came at the end of one live concert performance. The music's crescendo was intense and heavenly bliss is the only way to express what I felt. Then there was a fierce standing ovation, which took the joy to a level beyond words.

- Even in this world, when you are in a crowd, and a standing ovation breaks out, you can feel the crowd's emotion. The emotional swell can bring people to tears.

The difference is that in the 3D state, your nerves and emotions are on the low end of a scale of 1-10. In a high-dose session, all the insulation is stripped off the wires, and your nerves and emotions are closer to an 8 or 9/10. During the standing ovation, I could feel the emotion of every single person who was cheering, whistling, and applauding. That experience of thousands of vibratory emotions all erupting in my field was the most intense thing I have ever felt.

- Finally, the experience of being in the heavenly bliss state came with two strong emotions. The first was the feeling of WOW. It is so awe-inspiring. The second emotion was one of overwhelming gratitude for getting into a mystical state not once but twice. Certainly, I said Wow and Thank you 25 times during the experience.

The understanding of focusing on the music to elevate oneself supports the famous NDE experience of Harvard neurologist Dr. Eben Alexander. In 2008, he had an experience where he was shown the various levels of reality from the lower earthworm view to the highest realm, which he called "the core."

What moved him from level to level was music, and the movement upward was initiated by focusing on the level. He wrote about being in the lower realm and wishing to return to the higher levels:

I found myself wishing for the Spinning Melody to return. After an initial struggle to recall the notes, the gorgeous music, and the spinning ball of light-emitting, it blossomed into my awareness. They cut, once again, through the jellied muck, and I began to rise

into the worlds above. I slowly discovered that to know and to be able to think of something is all that one needs to move towards it. To think of the Spinning Melody was to make it appear, and to long for the higher worlds was to bring me there. The more familiar I was with the higher worlds above, the easier it was to return to it. I accomplished this back-and-forth movement from the muddy darkness of the realm of the earthworm's-eye view to the green brilliance of the Gateway and into the black but holy darkness of The Core any number of times.[7]

Near the four-hour mark, I realized that I was now hearing the music instead of being in it. The plant medicine was wearing off. I tried to get swept up into the music with concentration, and it was tough to do. When I did, I would lose focus quickly. It was over.

While at the height of the experience, it is effortless to focus. It is almost impossible not to focus. There is no wandering voice chattering away as in meditation. It is like a magnet is forcing me to watch what I am being shown.

The last item of interest in Session #6 was the feeling of someone in the room. This happened twice and was caused by what appeared to be a noise right beside the bed. Once it just felt like someone was there, but the other times I was utterly sure someone was there and that they had turned the light on. I was completely startled, and my heart was racing.

I knew that there would be no one there if I looked, but I still struggled to break the focus on what was happening to lift the blindfold and peek out the right side. It was dark, and no one was there.

Session 7- Power, Control, and Humility

No, no, you're not thinking; you're just logical.
-**Niels Bohr**

As with all previous trips, I felt unnerved before the start. It is my ego-mind playing guardian again. This kind of beginning to the night usually leads me to apologize in the middle of the experience that I did not trust. Your mind *in* the state is not the same mind that is there *before* the state.

Going through this second-guessing gives me more empathy for people who need a guide to be with them. It would reduce the anxiety going in. Perhaps it would allow one to go deeper. I am looking at trying this to test the model.

As with previous experiences, I go in with the understanding that nothing inside my consciousness can hurt me and that I must own the experience, trust, let go, and be open.

I took the medicine and started meditating with my Muse headband, as in Session #6. This time my mind wandered more as I heard the rainfall instead of the birds singing.

The meditation was 15 minutes, but I did not even get that far as the mushrooms' effects were taking over. This was the fastest onset ever. Later, I determined that this was from taking 250 mg of niacin three hours earlier. Niacin is like rocket fuel when mixed with psilocybin.

Quickly, I shut off the Muse and struggled to get set up. This was tricky as the physical world skills were already falling apart. I started to become disoriented. The dose was high, and soon I would be unable to do much.

Because of these disorienting effects, I had trouble setting up the music, the headset and finding the blindfold. Under the covers with the music, I knew that the disorientation, intense physical, sensory overload, and confusion would disappear. I would then go to the still quiet state of the other world-the bubble.

This did occur. It took maybe two minutes under the covers for the chaos to lift and for me to drift into the psilocybin world.

It started the same as other sessions with the colored, psychedelic patterns. In this session, I could actually see some of the shapes people talk about, but the bright fluorescent colors only outlined the figures, and it did not last long. Stanislov Grof, the Czech-born psychiatrist, stated that these structures are only a phase you go through as you go deeper.

That makes total sense as I only see them initially, and then they are gone.

I had expected to continue with the theme from Session #6, but it was not to be. Whatever the intelligence is behind these experiences, it seems to come up with a different plotline each time, almost like the mind does with dreams. This session would be darker, and that is not to mean bad. It was just a different spectrum of reality.

I hoped to focus on the music again and be lifted into the heavenly bliss state. I focused on the music, and nothing happened. It seemed I was not quite in enough, so I tried later and was still unable.

The music was important in this experience as it has been in all my sessions. It was just being used in a powerful but different way. As always, they seemed to be playing with the music at one point in the session. That is because the right music appears at precisely the right time to drive the emotion. At one critical point, I was taken to a climax experience and was stunned at how the music helped lift and move the experience. When the song ended, there was a silence, and I just vibrated in the stillness.

Seconds later, another commercial came on. It was just like watching TV when they break for a commercial when you are on the edge of your seat. I said, "I would applaud, but I don't want to move."

I stated that the most potent music drivers are the crescendos that elevate whatever emotion they are driving. In this session, I learned that this is not entirely true. The standing ovations are mega-drivers as all the people's emotion seems to mix with the high emotional state of the experience and send it off the charts.

In Session #7, I again heard the standing ovation and was overwhelmed. It was not the same experience as Session #6, but I forget what happened. The song name is a fit for the psilocybin trip. It is called Gracias a la Vida from Mercedes Sosa – Thanks to life.[8]

As the experience was starting, I knew that it was not going to be heavenly this time. There was a feeling that told me this, and as the experience went along, it manifested. Anyone unfamiliar with this state would probably be freaking out in fear right about now.

Because memories in sessions disappear so quickly after, I can only write a few of them down. This is made worse by the fact that I did not audio record much. In the experience, I thought that "they" did not want me to record.

I was being shown something, and it was so enthralling that I could not talk and watch it simultaneously. I would start to record and then not say anything as I concentrated on what I was sensing.[6] I would try again minutes later, but the same thing would happen. They wanted me to shut up and sense what they were showing.

The sensing part is bizarre and inexplicable to those who have not experienced it. It is entirely impossible to turn away

---

[6] As I mentioned in previous sessions, I really don't see anything except for a bit of psychedelic colors outlining shapes as I enter the field, and I only see that when I concentrate on them. Everything comes through sensation and when you give it a name there is a sense of resonance that this is true.

from watching. It could be compared to completely focused meditation where no outside thoughts are flowing in. There is only one thing, and I am reticent and motionless as I watch.

I have no idea what I was being shown. It did not make any sense. There were no words to describe it, except it had something to do with how things are created. The ideas of complexity, power, and ineffability came to mind. Even though it was probably my idea, I sensed they were saying, "just try and explain this." This was another reason I stopped taping, as what I was experiencing was beyond words. I would sense one intricate illustration of some process then would just think, Wow, but I have no idea what I had just seen. Then there would be another process, and again I would have no understanding or words for it, so the audio stayed off, and I felt good taking it all in. I can express that when things have formed, the emotions and feelings go in simultaneously. The creation comes out of a powerful and dark, slowly rotating mass.

Act 1

I sensed from the beginning that this would not be a joyful, blissful experience. It was a mystical state of revealing the power, control, and magnificence of the universe and its creative force.

When this feeling came up, I remembered to own the experience and open up and learn from what would be shown.

The first not-feeling thing that illustrated the lower mystical state I was in came when the background was illuminated. Suddenly, a shadow started coming across and blocking out the light. Whatever it was, it had a straight edge, almost like a piece of paper was moving in front of the light. This seemed to be happening higher up in my vision, at the top of a room.

I do remember the object that hovered over my body. It was black against black, so I just sensed it. What it appeared to be was a giant, flat object like the Phoenix Lights craft.[7]

The object was maybe one inch over my body as it slowly crossed over me. It was ominous, but I was not scared. I was certainly aware that I was helpless and thought any novice would lose it if this happened during their first experience.

The object had a field attached to it. It was creating immense pressure on my body as it went over. There was intense pressure on my upper chest. I thought maybe they were doing the "you're dying" thing again. I concentrated as the pressure increased and the object continued to move over from left to right. I was thinking, "Wow, is that thing ever close."

Looking back, that may have been what it was all about. It may have been a show of power and control.

---

[7] The Phoenix Lights craft was reported flying over Phoenix 100 feet off the ground and some people described the silent triangle object to be a mile or more in size.

Act 2

The next thing I can recall was another display of the power and control behind whatever reality is. As mentioned above, it was utterly incomprehensible, and so I couldn't record it. One scene would appear. It would be replaced with a second and then a third. I lay quietly and watched. I did not understand anything. I just felt the emotion and felt the sense of tremendous power and control by whatever was putting on the display.

Act 3

This is the part of the experience where the message comes in. I was not told anything directly. There was no voice in the clouds talking to me.

As I am trying to develop an idea of what the message or concept of this lesson is, it resonates within me. That gives me the sense that the concept is correct.

Then every time I think about it, I feel a resonance and sense of certainty. I interpret a message to me from the field. In thinking of ultimate reality, the teacher and I within the psilocybin experience are probably the same.

This was the same process used when I had my two noetic downloads in 2012 and 2017. There was a resonance when I thought about the right idea. This is described as an *objective reality* in the characteristics of a mystical state:

Without a discernible identity comes a sense of greater "objectivity," as though you are experiencing a much more intricate and profound reality. Everything does not just feel perfect; everything is innately perfect.

Here are the messages I got. There was a tremendously severe atmosphere surrounding them that came with intense emotion.

1. While viewing some sort of presentation about how powerful *the force* is behind the universe, I got the idea more than one time, "I defy you to explain on paper what you are seeing." Realizing I could not, I stopped talking into the audio recorder. There was nothing to say.

2. After being overwhelmed with what I was shown, I sensed the message, "you have not got a clue as to what is going on. You only think you do because you think you are smart." I was so totally overwhelmed at how complicated everything seemed to be. When I thought, "You have not got a clue!" There was a resonance. I kept repeating it, but during the event, it seemed like they kept looping the message along with intense emotions that come with the feeling of how insignificant I am in comparison to what is displayed in front of me.

3. Then I was told, "You are just a piece of shit and do not know it." Again, I felt about myself considering what I was viewing, and with it, there was a resonance. This feeling of insignificance is part of many mystical states. Usually, the analogy is that the experiencer feels like a

grain of sand on a beach compared to the magnificent universe. Again, I came to the session with this line in my head, as I felt enormously insignificant at that moment.

4. The final message was most dramatic and may also have been pulled from my mind. I thought I should surrender and pee myself like a dog in front of his master." I sensed an image of my dog doing that in the past. When scolded about something, my little dog Squishy would crouch down in front of me, lower his head and start peeing. It was a sign of complete surrender.

I immediately did the same thing, which may come as a surprise to some, but it is not. In almost all ayahuasca experiences, people experience vomiting and diarrhea. It is seen as a sign of purging the body and making the body clean for the lesson.

People who use Morning Glory seeds as a psychoactive plant will report vomiting, and many who are doing psilocybin will also vomit. (I maintain that if one keeps entirely still during the session, this will not happen.) This *surrender* was described in one psilocybin experience related by Roland Griffiths at Johns Hopkins:

I felt myself instinctively taking on the posture of prayer in my head. I was on my knees, hands clasped in front of me, and I bowed to this force. I wasn't scared or threatened in any way. It was more about reverence. I was showing my respect. I was humbled and honored to be in this presence. This presence was a feeling, not something I saw or heard. I only felt it, but it felt more real than any reality I have experienced. And it was a familiar place too. One I had felt before. It was when I surrendered to this that I felt like I let go.9

The strange thing about this wetting myself experience is that nothing in the experience stopped. It did not skip a beat. It was almost like it said, "no need for a clean-up in aisle six. Come and see what is in aisle seven."

Within seconds I had forgotten what had happened and the lesson continued unabated. There was no sense of time, but I would guess this happened at least an hour before it was over.

I had surrendered, and it was okay.

5. The last message came a bit later, and again it came out of my head. It was an analogy to explain the power and seriousness with which the creative process seemed to be conducted. The idea I got was "they are playing with loaded guns." This seemed terrific and funny, and I sensed the intelligence thought it was funny too. I said I would tell people that they are up against a force with loaded guns. The idea that this notion would be left with people is respecting *the force*. It has the power, which you, with your ego, only think you have.

When the messages came to me, they kept repeating in my head along with the emotions. I said, "Ok, I got the message. I understand." I thought this would end it, but the loop of the message and emotions started again. It was almost as if the training required hammering this concept into my head twenty times until there is nothing except a complete surrender.

Looking Back

Looking back, this experience fits most, if not all, of the classic characteristics of a mystical experience. These states were described by Alan Watts as:

> *[Mystical experiences are] those peculiar states of consciousness in which the individual discovers himself to be one continuous process with God, with the Universe, with the ground of Being, or whatever name he may use by cultural conditioning or personal preference for the ultimate and eternal reality.*

What I experienced was an extraordinarily neutral and tremendously powerful force. It was busy creating as it had done for eternity. The process was very orderly, and I was just there observing in a state of total awe.

- **Conscious Unity** – I was in union with everything around me. From time to time, I would sense "Grant," but he was over there doing something. This would be only momentary, like "there he is," and Grant would be gone again.
- Another characteristic of a mystical experience was described by Dr. Roland Griffith, who runs the

psilocybin research department at Johns Hopkins University, as a "**deeply felt positive mood: joy, ecstasy, blessedness, peace, tenderness, gentleness, tranquility, awe.**"

Awe was at the top of my list. Ecstasy was second. The day after this I experienced the "deeply felt positive mood."

- There Is **No Time or Space**. I was surprised when it was over that my trip lasted 4.5 hours. From time to time during the experience, I would sense "Grant" and when I concentrated, some sense of time would come back as to where I was and what I was doing, but only if I focused. When I stopped concentrating, I would flow back into the experience.

- **Gratitude-** Even though there was no bliss or heavenly state this time, I felt what is described as "ecstatic feelings stemming from an immense sense of gratitude." "As the definition continues, "it is an overwhelming sense of awe at 'your' (now non-existent) insignificance in comparison to the vastness of existence." That was the critical part of the message of this experience, which I will relate to later. I felt very honored and grateful for the experience as it ended.

- **Life is seen as sacred-** This was part of the experience, but the sacredness came from the understanding that life's creation is extraordinarily complex and beyond our comprehension. The revelation was very moving, coming with an extreme emotional feeling that embedded itself and was still there after the memory of the details had faded. As the definition says, there is a "new sense of respect for the sacredness of life that allows you to be here."

- The next characteristic of a mystical state is "**paradox after paradox**" (e.g., something is both light/dark, here/absent, human/divine, limited/eternal). This was a darker experience, but it was the same mystical state that created bliss. All experiences are equal, and all bring lessons about how reality works. There is no dark and light, or good and evil. There is just experience. This is one of the almost impossible principles to explain to someone who has not felt it.

- **The Experience Is Indescribable** – This is an absolute understatement related to Session #7. There were no words that could ever describe what I was being shown. I even resonated with a thought in my head which said with laughter, "I defy you to try and describe what you are seeing." I just gave up and watched instead of describing what I see in the recorder.

- **The Experience Is Temporary** – Life goes on. The illusionary reality seeps back in. This feeling began the moment I took off the blindfold and turned off the music. I could almost feel the physical world flowing back; it was almost like waking up in the morning. Something changes inside you, and that is undoubtedly true.

- **The Experience Is Life-Changing** –I spent the morning today, the day after my trip, wandering the streets in a calm daze, thinking about the few things I remember from the trip, and feeling the emotions of this lesson continues to be with me.

Session 8 – The Hooker

There are some things so serious you have to laugh at them.
                                                    -Neils Bohr

Act 1 – The Dancing Bears

As I write up this experience the morning after, I am still laughing. It has been four hours of constant laughter. Yes, whatever intelligence I encountered has a fantastic sense of humor. With what I was given, I could do a stand-up comedy routine on stage in New York.

The entire trip lasted four hours. The audiotape was 3 hours and 47 minutes long, which means a lot was happening, and it started early. Before the session, I had resolved not to talk much this time, but that did not happen.

Within minutes of the start, I felt intense pressure on my chest. I always looked for what the theme would be. At first, I thought this session would be on intensity. It started so intensely that it was no surprise as this was the highest dose I had ever used.

117

After four-hours in, I pleaded for more, and it was like they said, "No, the show is over. We are closing the curtain." I thought it would be longer as this time I was up to taking nearly six grams. I went in as always with a simple intention, to sit quietly and watch what they show me. I do not move a muscle and am riveted at the impressions given to me.

I have a stringent protocol for getting into the field, so there are no surprises. As I was eating my six grams, I realized that this was the most challenging part of the experience. I use cherry yogurt, which I once loved but cannot even look at anymore.

As the trip began, the voice of a West Jet stewardess rang in my head as he demonstrated the safety rules "Please fasten your seatbelts. We are about to go very, very fast."

The Universe did not let me down. It was like the curtain opened and the show began. It almost didn't wait for me to get under the covers. Out came the dancing bears. I found the session so captivating and enthralling I could not look away. There is no wandering mind happening as when I try to meditate.

The following analogy may help explain the difference between lower and higher dose trips, where I took between 3 -6 grams. The 3-gram experience is like a hockey game where one team scores 5 minutes in and the final score is 1-0. The 6-gram experience is like an 8-7 game where one team ties it up with two goals in the last two minutes and wins it 30 seconds into overtime.

After the whole thing was over, the joke came to me that they were lying in wait for me this night. Luckily, I got the entire experience on the recording, and it was more real than the real world, even though some of it sounds insane. On the recording, I said, "I am just describing what I am seeing and sensing, and it appears utterly real. If this was a hallucination, then all of life is hallucination because there is absolutely nothing different."

The session started with fluorescent colors. They were mostly yellow, purple, and some green, and the whole session started with a red glow coming from the right. The colors seemed to bring some brightness into the dark. Yet there was no light. On the recording, I said, "there is darkness and light, but no light." It reminded me of the light reported by people who have been on a UFO who say there was a bright light, but there didn't appear to be any source of it.

The lights to me were like clouds that the plane must pass through to get to the proper altitude. Usually, I do not perceive much of this, and that may be because I am not interested in it, so I do not pay much attention when it happens.

Just as the colorful images were ending, I had a bizarre déjà vu experience. It was powerful and was the first time I had ever experienced this phenomenon. It was not a moment of a déjà vu feeling but an event that went on for 10 minutes. I sensed that déjà vu was an actual thing. It was like it seemed to be a substance. No event was explicitly recalled, and two different songs were involved, so it was not the song that triggered it.

As I drifted deep into the field, I became aware of how the mind struggles to find words to explain what is going on. This time an analogy popped into my mind that seemed to describe what is happening. When you start to daydream as someone is talking to you, they notice it and attempt to pull you out of the dream. But you are enjoying watching the dancing bears in your mind so much that you forget how to find your way back to hear what they are saying.

Act 2 – The Bathroom Again

One drawback as the experience began, I had to go to the bathroom the minute I laid down. I became frustrated as this is a reoccurring problem. It is tough to let go of the experience when this occurs.

I tried to evade the bathroom problem in this session. I did not drink anything since noon that day, which was 7 hours earlier. It did not make any sense. I broke the bubble and angrily when to the bathroom, where nothing happened. Back to bed, and the same thing happened. I held off for 10 minutes, and as a commercial came on, I returned to the bathroom, where I was able to come up with a little.

Thinking this solved it, I got back into bed and again had to go to the bathroom. At that point, I said No more. For the whole four-hour trip, the sensation remained. After I came out of it, I was awake for two more hours and still had to go even though it had now been 13 hours since I had drunk anything.

The two-bathroom trips did reestablish the idea of breaking the bubble. When you are quiet, with a blindfold, with a headset with music, and under the covers, that setting provides for a blissful state where you can calmly surrender and watch the show.

During my bathroom interruptions, I recorded how disorienting it is outside of the bubble and then how happy I was to be back in the setting under my covers.

The next day it occurred to me what might be going on. When I do the high dose, I notice the floating sensation followed by an intense vibration that seems to be in every cell of my body. I concluded that this vibration was causing the bathroom problem. It was vibrating the prostate, which caused the bathroom sensation.

I went to google and searched psilocybin and prostate to research this, figuring that others must have experienced the same problem. Maybe they could tell me how to avoid the problem.

I read one man commenting, but his problem was a bit different, saying he was "peeing frequently but peeing is hard to do, and I feel like my bladder is full." The search also yielded an article describing research into mushrooms and prostate cancer.

Recent developments in mushrooms as an anti-cancer therapeutic remedy show:

> *The active components in mushrooms responsible for conferring anti-cancer potential are lentinan, krestin, hispolon, lectin, calcaelin, illudin S,*

psilocybin, Hericium polysaccharide A and B (HPA and HPB), ganoderic acid, schizophyllan, laccase, etc.[10]

It makes one wonder what the connection here is, as there are so few studies using psilocybin.

Act 3- A Message for the Skeptics

The way the information comes to me is through sensing. This contact modality is no different than any other. The only difference is this one will determine how far into the non-local field you go. Based on many hours in the field, I know that a noetic flow state is created there.

I am talking into the recording device and explaining what I am seeing. I suddenly resonate with something that I have said. The stronger the resonance, the more real the idea appears to be for me.

Knowing that these recordings would sound crazy, whatever intelligence I was dealing with gave me a couple of comeback lines. One was told to me back in Chapter 7, but they seemed to add a line to it in this session.

In Session #7, the message was, "You are just a piece of doodoo (actually sensed a more explicit term) that thinks that you understand how reality works. In reality, you haven't got a clue."

In Session #8, this insight was clarified and expanded upon saying, "You are arrogant and ignorant little pieces of doodoo, who think you understand how reality works when you have got no clue. The worst part is that you don't even realize that they are arrogant and ignorant pieces of doodoo that think they understand reality when they don't have a clue. Is that not true?"

It is true. It became even more true when I discovered months later that Terence McKenna got the same message:

> *The mushroom told me nobody knows jack shit about what is going on.*

The messages I have received from the intelligence behind the psilocybin can be very blunt. When I first heard this one directed at me, I thought, "How could you say that? I am such a nice guy."

This was an amusing session. The Universe can be blunt but funny. I was given the sense of humanity as the "Twitter guy." The scene goes like this:

> *I am the Twitter guy. Have you ever heard of Twitter? I'm on it. I am a brilliant genius on Twitter. I am the Twitter guy. Ask me anything. I will tell you how it works. I will do it in 280 characters and be done in 2 minutes. Ask me anything. I am the twitter guy.*

Other people who have received this blunt message from the intelligence include both Dennis and Terence McKenna. Dennis McKenna had done ayahuasca in Brazil and realized that we were destroying the rain forest and felt he had to do something. He became panicked about the situation when he received the message:

Ayahuasca tells me, 'you monkeys only think you're running the show,' but it's co-evolution. The plants are running the show.

Then there is the statement made by Terence McKenna, which I am sure he got from the intelligence. It has to do with the arrogant little pieces of doodoo who think they have it all figured out when in reality, they are just making up stories. McKenna stated:

Do you know what the straight people are selling? They're selling that the universe sprang from nothing, for no reason instantly. Well, now I submit to you that this is the limit case for credulity. If you believe that, my family owns a bridge over the Hudson River to sell you very cheaply. The idea that the universe could spring instantly from nothing for no reason is they just saying, "test them with this, Charlie. If they'll buy that, what wouldn't they buy, for crying out loud?

And this is tenant One of science. Essentially, what science says is, 'Give us one free miracle - one free miracle - and we can just work with that. We can unfold that, invest that, fold it back, expand it, comment on it you know, copy it, verify it.'

*Well, so then, apparently, you get one free **miracle when you play this game.**[11]*

Although this may seem a bit harsh for a universal loving force, it is just a recurrence of one of the classic, mystical experience characteristics.

The discovery during the mystical experience is that you (now non-existent) are insignificant compared to the vastness of existence.

Although the person inside the experience will accept this, the skeptic looking in does not accept the status of *insignificance*. Skeptics are generally stuck in the "ego" of the left brain and think they are brilliant and can describe everything in the universe, which is considered insignificant, random noise.

One example of this would-be Professor Philip Jolly, who in 1974 told his student, later Nobel Laureate and father of quantum physics Max Planck, not to go into physics because "in this field, almost everything is already discovered, and all that remains is to fill a few unimportant holes."

Another example would be Charles H. Duell, who was the Commissioner of the US Patent Office. He stated in 1902, "everything that can be invented has been invented."

Act 4 – Enter the Hooker

This must go down as the wildest in all my psilocybin experiences. Like everything else in these temporary altered states of consciousness, words cannot accurately describe what was happening. Also, this experience fits the mystical state in that it had a sense of greater "objectivity," as though I was experiencing a much more intricate and profound reality

This event was a display of the workings of the Universe. I had been shown this universal reality in Session #7. They delivered it to me and defied me to write it down. This second display was much more spectacular and moving.

Here is the transcript of the recording as I'm describing the event. This started very early, at 41:00 minutes into the session. In this segment, the reader will also begin to understand why the chapter is called a *Hooker*. I thought that the Universe showing off to me had happened later in the session, but it started here very early. (The transcript is choppy in parts because I am continually trying to find the words to explain something that cannot be labeled).

They just basically told me that they would lead me through it.

(Whispering) Absolutely beyond words. I'm in it. Was in it with the music.

(Still whispering) You forget who you are. This has absolutely shattered my view of what reality is. It has turned my view of reality right on its head.

(Whispering) Shattered my view. Unbelievable.

Thank you.

Thank you.

I don't even know where to start. You forget that you are in it. You're not talking. Thank you. Oh my God. I had no idea. You have no idea! They are playing this music. Thank you. Oh my God.

Ohhhhh. Ohhh. Thank you.

I was shown it.

Ohhhh. Thank you. Thank you.

Thank you. Thank you. Thank you.

Ohhhh. Ohhhhh. (Laughs) Thank you.

Thank you. Thank you.

Ahhh. Thank you.

Ahhh, the music. Thank you.

Thank you.

Ahhh, thank you.

Ahhh, thank you.

I was shown how the Universe operates.

Here it comes again. They are going to show it again.

They are going to show me again. Thank you.

Ahhhh, this is déjà vu. Thank you.

My idea of how reality works is shattered. Thank you.

No idea.

Ohhhh, thank you.

Ohhhh, the music is playing

(Laughs) It's just (pause) Thank you.

Unbelievable.

It's like trying to describe what's happening here

The feeling is (laughs); it is like it is showing off.

My theory of reality has been set on its head.

I don't even know where to start.

Thank you.

As usual, I am sure they are playing with the music, or Johns Hopkins has the music down pat. They are playing with music.

Thank you. I had no idea.

It is like it is dragging me into it. I am in it.

It is showing off. It is like it is saying, "Watch this!"

I feel so honored. Sooo honored to see this!

So, honored! My view of reality is absolutely shattered.

I had no idea.

The vibration. Vibration. You lose it. The color. The vibration. You are in this.

People have no clue.

It's almost like they were waiting for me to come along to show…

I forget, ah ah… (looking for words)

There is intense pressure in the chest. I am feeling like I have to go to the bathroom.

The music, like, they control the music. Do you think they control the music?

Oh, get out of here, little girl! (Talking to the force)

Hopefully, the tape recorder is working.

Ohhhh my God, the vibration is, (inaudible) surrender!

You might as well turn the tape recorder off.

You sort of remember who you are. It is hard to describe.

Try to stay focused.

My sense of reality is completely shattered.

Hmmmm. When you start talking about it, you move out (meaning out of the field and back into hallucinatory reality)

Ah, it's dragging me back in here.

This is incredible

As is evident, the experience brought a sense of gratitude and a reason for not deserving the opportunity to experience such a miracle. Both are characteristics of the mystical experience (see Appendix 1). Also included was another aspect of it; a new sense of respect for the sacredness of life that allows one to be here.

This incredible event was highlighted by the fact that the "intelligence" or "field" or "force" had a female essence to it. This was the first time I had felt this, but it did not last.

After the intelligence showed me the Universe's operation, I was surprised to see that it started showing off. It repeated flaunted itself. It was nothing I could see. It was a sense of power, intelligence, and beauty that was coming through the music. As with other messages, the message's emotion and feeling would become more potent as the music crested.

The source appeared to be female, and the feeling it instilled in me was like beholding a stunningly beautiful woman. This is the kind of allure that has caused many men to risk their careers, marriages, or even lives to be with this woman for even just a few hours.

This state is very similar to situations I run into when talking to people who have encountered being on a UFO. They will tell me what happened at some point will say "he" or "she." (Usually, it is a he.)

When the person completes their story, I usually ask them if they had clothes. Usually, the answer is No.

Then I ask if they noticed if the being had any sex organs. The person will think and almost always reply, No.

Then I ask them how they knew it was a male or a female if they did not see sex organs. They will pause again and all give the same answer. "I just knew it was male or female. I do not know how, but I knew what it was."

This would indicate that the being gives off some sort of field or vibe that can be read as either male or female. That would explain what I experienced. There was nothing visible that told me it was a female, but I would bet all the poker chips that it was. It was exceedingly obvious.[8]

The Universal power was provoking envy or admiration and appeared to be showing off. The closest analogy would be a prostitute displaying on a street corner looking for business. It was almost like it was calling out, "Hey, little boy. Check this out." Even though there was nothing sexual about what it was

---

[8] This would lead to an important clue in the UFO community about what they are dealing with regarding UFOs. Unfortunately, some UFO researchers are consumed with UFO sightings and things that might be nuts and bolts related to the phenomenon that they can make benefit from financially.

doing, I was a bit embarrassed and asked it to stop, but it did not.

As crude as some people may think this whole story is, the awe that it inspired fits right into one of the nine traits of a mystical experience that are occasioned when people do high dose psilocybin:

> *In this profound state of being, you feel that life is full of beauty and sacredness – yet this feeling is not subjective but is instead an objective phenomenon that is outside yourself.*[12]

After a while of this bizarre display to attract attention, I effectively started to laugh uncontrollably and played along. I do not recall what they were showing me but, on the recording, I kept repeating that:

1) It appeared to be a female force.

2) It was showing off, but I do not remember anything except the music was involved.

3) I just kept yelling Bravo! and repeated over, and over that, I believed it was showing off.

4) No one would be able to understand what I was sensing, and I probably could not convey it.

5) This went on for over an hour.

6) I kept laughing as it cycled through its show.

7) It appeared the music was controlled, but in reality, the intense emotion involved made it feel like the music was part of the experience. (Johns Hopkins, I believe, has a specific type of music at this point in the list on purpose.)

8) Once again, I do not think I actually saw anything.

9) I was in a complete state of ecstasy.

10) At one time during the high point, I felt and described a feeling of unconditional love. This is the first time in my life I can recall such a feeling.

11) The experience had the mystical-state situation of "overwhelming magnitude of emotions." That description does not even come close to what I experienced. All the emotions were positive, and I have never laughed so hard for so long. The reason for the laughter was that *the force* kept showing off and would not stop.

12) At several points, I state that I was talking to someone or something, and it appeared to be female.

After 2.5 hours, I took a break to go to the bathroom. When I got back into the field, the female had now taken on a male essence. I could still sense a show of majesty, but my excitement had dropped way down.

Act 5- Unconditional Love

When a person does psilocybin, much of what transpires is forgotten. This leads some researchers to recommend not doing it. The unconditional love experience was one of the things that I forgot until I got a brief recollection the day after. I realized that I had felt unconditional love, which is also described by many experiencers in alien encounters and near-death experiences.

During my research, while writing the book *Contact Modalities,* I found that people can use many completely different techniques to get into the non-local field. I tried many of the methods without success. One of the ones I attempted was lucid dreaming, where you can train yourself to pick up on dream clues and then become lucid in the dream state. I tried every technique but with zero success. I even tried pills that had been used in the Stanford University lucid dream lab with great success. They did not work for me.

The idea is that you can interact with the universe while in this lucid state and ask anything you want. Supposedly, an answer will come. I was always ready for the moment I would have a breakthrough and would ask to have the experience of unconditional love.

Luckily, even though I forgot the experience, I could go back to the recording and hear that it happened.

Like other experiences, I felt like the luckiest person in the world; I kept saying, Thank you! and wondered why I would be allowed to have this experience, which most people don't get.

Unconditional love is listed as one of the traits of mystical experiences that are brought on by high-dose psilocybin. In a study published by Johns Hopkins University in 2008 called, *Mystical-Type Experiences Occasioned by Psilocybin Mediate the Attribution of Personal Meaning and Spiritual Significance 14 Months Later,* one participant described encountering this unconditional love:

> *The understanding that in the eyes of God - all people...were all equally important and equally loved by God. I have had other transcendent experiences; however, this one was important because it reminded and comforted me that God is truly and unconditionally loving and present.*[13]

Act 6- A Conversation with The Force

> *I have a message for you from the Guardians. They want you to know that the message is in the music.*
> **-Message to me from experiencer Chris Bledsoe 2014**

> *I ain't never wrote nothin. Those songs was float'n in the air, and I just pulled them down.*
> **-Bob Monroe, the father of modern Bluegrass music**

As mentioned previously; I don't *see* anything or hear any voices. Everything is sensed through vibration and emotion. I interpret the messages as ideas that I think of and then resonate as accurate.

This may sound like a touchy-feely thing with no substance, but I can assure the reader that what I am sensing is as real as anything in 3D reality. It may be even more realistic because it comes with extreme emotion that is not present in our everyday hallucinatory reality.

When I listened to the recording of this part, I was horrified. I sounded crazy. Thinking back to the event, I said, "No, I remember this, and it was as real as the real world."

I turned the recorder on, and No, I sounded crazy. I concluded that I would vote with the absurd conclusion people.

People who know me believe I am reserved and quiet unless I am in a lecture or interview. Here, I was alone, and I was more excited than anyone I have ever seen.

I was swearing a lot, which was a bit embarrassing. I decided to edit that all out and then realized that there was so much swearing it would take forever. I would destroy the tape and keep the memory. Later thinking back on it, I realized that unless you have Terence McKenna's vocabulary, there is a lack of accurate words to describe the most fantastic experience of one's life. That's where the swear words came in.

This part of the session's most significant focus was the conversation I was having with the Universe. It didn't help that I am defending how crazy it will sound on the recording, but it is happening in real-time with no elements of hallucination of the dream.

I was continually laughing as I engaged with whatever it was. I was yelling Bravo! over and over as it showed off. (I was still laughing through the next day). It was VERY STRANGE but genuine.

I kept talking about the music on the tape but didn't talk about what I had been shown. I do recall a moment as I came out of what they were showing me. It was like coming out of a tunnel or portal, and I could tell I had just been somewhere very strange as returning to the 3D world; there was a contrast at the boundary. As I looked back, I could see where I had just been and thought, "What the hell was that?"

What did I see? I have no clue. There are no words to describe it, even if I remembered. Whatever it was, it got me very excited. Whatever it was left as quickly as I was shown it.

As I listened to the audio, the constant excited talk about the music became overwhelming. The music fit the feeling so well that "they" had to be playing with (interfering with) the music.

The communication came through the music. I am sure that is how it was working.

Like every session before this one, I became one with the music and had a powerful feeling that it was being manipulated. That is because the music reflects what I am thinking and experiencing. This is hard to explain to people who have not experienced it because no analogy in the physical world illustrates it.

The best example of that music that was mentioned before is *Gracias a la Vida* by Mercedes Sosa on the *Johns Hopkins playlist,* which has a standing ovation at the end. In our ordinary 3D reality, being in a crowd performing a standing ovation can be a very emotional experience. At the height of a trip, it takes the individual into a state that can only be labeled as *bliss* or *rapture.*

I don't recall what I was shown, but a bell did go off later when I heard Joe Rogan talk about turning on a tape recorder post-trip after doing 5-MeO DMT. He stated that:

> *...as I am trying to recount what happened, I could feel my ego trying to retake the situation in a way that might impress you with my ability to describe things. As a professional comedian, I was aware that you are saying things that are pleasing to people, so they get excited about hearing you talk. I was very aware of that when I was doing it. I am trying to explain things that are not possible to explain because the words we were using were all invented for a world that does not exist in the DMT world.*[14]

As I looked back on the excitement of the experience, I was selling the encounter big time. The strange part of that performance was the ego's *bad trip*, which was scared going in but was now taking credit for everything that had occurred.

As with many things I have witnessed in high-dose sessions, the message that was delivered was looped. It just keeps driving the message and connected emotion until I am pleading for it to stop. In this session, I found this looping experience very funny.

Dr. Bill Richards, who created the playlist used during psilocybin sessions at Johns Hopkins University, described the role of music as follows:

> *My preference is not to use either the words 'augmenting' or 'the psychedelic experience.' Profound states of consciousness can occur in silence, and there are many discrete states of awareness that can make up a particular 'psychedelic experience' (or*

series of 'experiences'). With adequate dosage, I do not feel that the music 'causes' particular experiences; rather, it supports and undergirds the experiential flow, as the content is emerging for the particular person.[15]

A study done on music and LSD showed a similar powerful connection:

Music is a classic means of evoking emotion, and like LSD, it has also been used as an adjunct to psychotherapy. Music has accompanied ceremonial use of psychedelics for many centuries, was a staple component in psychedelic-assisted psychotherapy in the 1950s and 1960s, and remains so today.

It has been proposed that listening to music during a psychedelic experience is useful for (1) encouraging the relinquishment of control, (2) facilitating emotional arousal and release, (3) promoting the occurrence of peak or spiritual-type experiences, (4) directing and/or structuring the experience, and (5) stimulating the imagination. Profound spiritual- or mystical-type experiences were reported by a majority of participants in a study with another psychedelic drug, psilocybin, while they listened to emotionally evocative music. This raises an important question: what is the role of music in producing such profound psychological experiences?[16]

In 2014, my friend, Chris Bledsoe, told me that he had received a message from the beings he was dealing with, and the message was for me. He told me that the Guardians wanted me to know that "the message was in the music."

At that time in my life, the message meant nothing to me as I did not listen to music and never have. Chris told me further that he thought Neil Young was part of the story about delivering the message, and because Young grew up in my city of Winnipeg, the synchronicity led me to check out the idea that "the message is in the music." That investigation led to a book I wrote called *Tuned in: The Paranormal World of Music.* It focused on musicians who received songs spontaneously, in dreams, and where they believed they were dealing with a force greater than themselves.

After this interaction with the music in Session #8, the message Chris had given me popped into my head. It sent shivers down my spine as I now knew the message was real.

Despite how powerful the music is, I got an insight into trying a high-dose session without the music. By doing this, I will be able to tell how much of a factor the music plays. At the end of Session #8, I would feel that the music almost overrides everything else, so it might be time to find out if there is something else outside the music.

Session 9 – Yell- Bravo! and Applaud Like Hell!!

In Chapter 8, I felt after listening to the audio recording that the music had dominated the whole session. Music does drive the experience, and that is a vital part of the event.

I and many others, like Michael Pollan, knew that part of the experience is being one with the music, which is something that must be experienced to be understood. Here is how Pollan described it:

> What happened then is I merged with this piece of music. I became one with this Yo-Yo Ma. I could almost feel the horsehair of the bow going over my skin. There was no space between me and this music. I was the music. It was an astonishing experience. It was ecstatic in the literal sense of my usual body.[17]

I knew from the story told by bestselling writer Michael Pollan that music can mess up what happens during a trip. He had used a female guide who rejected the *Johns Hopkins playlist* to use music she thought would work better. This is a bit like just wandering off into the forest instead of following the path that was created by the guide who had journeyed the road many times.

Pollan ended up in a computer world scene that he did not like, and after taking a bathroom break, he asked to have the music changed. She then put on a classical piece, and the experience turned positive.

A few days later, while walking in the park, I got an insight to do a session without music to see how it compared. I had reservations about wondering if anything significant would happen or if I would waste a week, but I thought I had to do this.

At the last moment, I chose to go with the music and record it. I had become addicted to music. I learned way more using this but remembered nothing except a few things. Most of what I am left with are feelings about the awe of the Universe and a vision I got which I thought related to the present situation in the United States.

At the end of Session #9, I felt that I had been shown more than any other session and felt like a changed individual.

Act 1 – The Start

What you focus on appears, and what you don't focus on just disappears like a dream. You can't get it back.

-Grant Cameron

As you move into the psychedelic field, you move through a layer of colors and shapes. It is almost like flying through clouds to get to cruising altitude.

I impatiently waited as things started. Since talking pulls the observer away, I was determined to speak as little as possible to allow me to go deeper into what I would be shown. The vibration was starting in my arms and then moving to my whole body. The vibration was potent, concentrated, and extremely high frequency, making it feel very smooth. I could almost feel the texture of it, which would have resembled silk. It had a female quality.

I waited for the colors to come, but there were NO COLORS. NO PATTERNS. NONE. I was incredibly pleased with this as it indicated to me that I was starting to be able to control the whole session by intention. I am not interested in colors or shapes and felt that I had some control, as I stopped them from appearing. I went straight into what hopefully would be a training session.

Just before that happened, I sensed someone in my room on my right and at the foot of the bed, and they had turned on the lights. I said, "It's not a bad sense, but it is as real as can be. An incredible sense that someone is in the room with me." It lasted for a couple of minutes and then went away. I did not look out to see what was happening.

Like previous sessions, the vibration became very intense, and I thought that the theme would be vibration, possibly, this time. Once again, the information, sensing, and emotion were coming through the music. As I got deeper and deeper, the sense of being One with the music increased, and I felt like it was being put into me through firstly a spot in the center of my chest and in a spot right above my third eye from some field that seemed to be less than an inch from my head.

Act 2- The Music Show

The beginning of the trip focused on music as that was on my mind. I understood a connection to the music that left me speechless. The message did not leave me behind. It was almost like the songs were alive and asking me not to cut them loose.

Even though the music did not dominate my trip like in Session #8, it put on a first-class show, like the songs trying to show me how important they were.

I was very eager to get into the field. Once in it, I felt like I was in an intense field vibrating and that the music was vibrating inside the larger field. The music carries emotion in its vibration.

Act 3 - Compassion

At one point, roughly three hours in, I was suddenly thrown into an emotional situation where I could feel the pain and loss of the whole world. Here is what I said as it was happening. It came during a song that fit the emotion of death and loss:

> *The feeling that I feel right now… they are showing me all the deaths of mankind. I can feel the pain and loss. I can feel the loss of all those people, but I would not have done it without the music (long pause.) You*

are literally dragged into the emotion, the tears, the sorrow. Whoever was right. Whoever was wrong, people cried. People cried. Whoever was right. Whoever was wrong, people cried? They left the loss. I feel an overwhelming feeling of the loss that the people felt. I can feel the loss. It's weird. So, if you have someone die, and you had that sense of loss. They are showing that to me right now as we speak. I am feeling the loss. I feel the loss. I am vibrating as the losses build. It is like the losses are coming one after another. I am observing them. It's okay. They are telling me, 'We feel the pain. We feel the pain. It's okay.' They are telling me, 'We feel the pain of people dying.' (whispering) They tell me, 'It's okay. It's okay.' They say, 'They know. They feel the pain.'

They feel the loss of people dying. They are saying, 'It will be okay.' It is still a magnificent Universe no matter what people do to it. It is still a magnificent Universe.

Act 4- The Vision

One thing that was heavily on my mind was the U.S. election, and they did show me some stuff there. At least, that is what I thought.

During this, I thought I was channeling, which made me uncomfortable as I have never sensed I would do such a thing. I have just recorded what I saw and felt in words.

The image I was shown many times during the session was a dark, nighttime ocean scene comparable to the inside of a hurricane. There were huge waves and swirling action. (The swirling was like a dark hurricane, but I knew it didn't mean there would be a hurricane.) I got the message (feeling) that this is just a natural process of the Universe and that there is no offense to whoever gets caught up in it.

It seemed to be aiming at the United States situation, where there's a tremendous amount of negative energy being put into the mix. This was shown to me as being similar to a hurricane with excess energy in the ocean because of high water temperatures. This energy builds and builds, and the cyclone is the mechanism that releases the energy. The message was, "We have to let off some steam. The energy has built up." It came with the idea that it was nothing personal.

I was told that the energy is building and will have to be released. As Edgar Cayce said, "Thoughts are things." On the other hand, people think thoughts are not things, and we can say anything we want. They believe that their thoughts immediately dissipate. The idea was that they do not dissipate; they build up at a critical high point, and then the excess energy must be released.

I was left with the feeling of an upcoming disaster that would arise from the energy being thrown around because of the election. I had a dark, foreboding sense that there would be some significant, dark event that would be part of the process of how the universe works. It was energy in and energy out and nothing personal. During this event, I was feeling the pain and suffering of all the people in the world. I kept saying, "I'm sorry. I'm so very sorry. That is all I can do."

When this was over, I got the message that we will rebuild after it is all over. Despite all the pain and sorrow, we will rebuild.

Coming out of it, I evaluated whether or not to make the vision public and decided against it.

I burped twice and realized that the stomachache I had had 24/7 for weeks already, was suddenly gone. It occurred to me that this might have been part of the dark swirling waters and the message that there is a lot of energy building up and it must be released.

I woke in the morning to discover that I did not have a stomachache for the first time in many months. Perhaps the swirling mass *was* my stomach, which was why they showed it to me, and maybe it had nothing to do with the United States. In my integration, I concluded that energy in and energy out was a fundamental law of the Universe, and it applied to all situations.

One week later, and my stomachache has not returned.

Act 5- Complexity

I have graduated kindergarten, and the lessons are becoming more strenuous and hard to grasp, so I will have to rely on the recording. One of the things I learned was that it appears and becomes real in the psilocybin world when you focus on something. When you take your focus away, it disappears. When I would pause to find the words to describe what I was sensing, what I wanted to talk about was gone entirely. Most of what I felt had disappeared. I hoped to be able to explain it in the recording.

On the audio, I explained this as being shown things in the here and now. You either focus on it, or you can see it disappear. Secondly, I noticed that it was hard to concentrate long enough to describe anything as the music's intensity dragged my focus away.

Unfortunately, it is hard to speak as my awareness became transfixed on the latest bobble I was shown. It is precisely like daydreaming, where you sort of pop out of what you were sensing. If I spoke during the daydream, I would have it on tape. Much would be lost.

Therefore, in a high-dose session, you should run an audio recorder, as you will remember extraordinarily little when it is over. Ethnopharmacologist Dennis McKenna even used this forgetting as a reason for people to try micro-dosing instead, as opposed to his brother Terence. The latter recommended a 5-gram hero dose while sitting in a dark room. In high-dose sessions, it is tough to bring back what you experienced into waking reality.

This may be why I still have no clue beyond the focus thing after tripping so many weeks in a row.

Act 6 – A Deep Sense of Awe

The force of the Universe had exhibited its power and grandeur. It was showing off again. Even the way they put it through the music was impressive and eerie. The musical piece would build and build, and I would sense the power and grandeur of the Universe. As the song came to the crescendo, I would be swept up into a sense of ecstasy which is tied into the vibration and overcome with a feeling of awe. The song would end, and there would be silence. Spotify would go to commercial. I thought, "How the hell do they do that?"

But the final part of the night was off the charts. Here is how I described it on tape:

> *Let me give you a sense of what happened at the end. No matter what kind of dose I take, it is over after four hours. I knew when I looked under the blindfold it would be 10 o'clock, and it was 10 o'clock. There was this grand finale song that was the end of the show. Here we go! The magnificence of the Universe. I am wrapped up in emotion, awe, and reverence. Then it stops, and it is like, 'That's four hours! Close the curtain'…. You go from totally in it to not in it at all.*

The only analogy I can think of that can describe this is if you are in the middle of a crowd that suddenly breaks into a standing ovation.

The message was that people are motivated, not by logic or facts, but by emotion. It seemed to indicate that this is happening in politics when people get a good feeling from a politician and are swept up without considering any other factors. The same might apply to falling in love, where people are swept up in emotion. When that emotion wears off, each partner wonders, "What was I thinking?" The point is that they were not thinking.

Act 7- Gratitude

One of the characteristics of a mystic experience is a sense of gratitude. That was apparent again in Session nine. My takeaway from this session was that all you can do is throw up your hands, yell Bravo! and applaud like hell. I am the luckiest person alive to have been shown all of this. Thank you! Thank you! Thank you!

Session 10 - Thank You

Act 1

I decide to change the strain of mushrooms for Session #10. In the catalogs, the descriptions for the various strains of magic mushroom say things like, "It is known to give one of the warmest visual and spiritual trips. It is an all-around and versatile mushroom," or "They are best known for their shamanistic properties, or spiritual effects rather than solely 'tripping.'"

This is strange because the common claim from the various university labs doing their research is that it is all just psilocybin, which becomes psilocin, which influences the brain's serotonin 2A receptor. The catalogs seem to imply that each type of mushroom brings its qualities to the experience. This is critical to the debate on whether one should use the actual product or the synthesized version.

I decided to use a mushroom described as "Known to be one of the strongest and hard-hitting. Expect deep shamanic experiences, vision quests, and an intense mystical experience. Not recommended for first-time users." The idea was to see if 1.5 grams of these powerful mushrooms would produce effects that I hadn't experienced during my first nine sessions. If there is a difference, it would mean that other substances in the mushrooms besides psilocybin influence what is experienced.

After taking the dose and waiting for about an hour, I got over the fear that these powerful mushrooms would cause trouble as the fearful write-up had warned, and since not much was happening. I decided to take a 0.5-gram booster that was sitting out on the desk.

I wanted to establish with this new mushroom strain that if it was indeed different from the Golden Teacher mushrooms that I had used previously. If the tryptamine alkaloid, known as psilocybin, causes the experience, then if one consumes the same dose of psilocybin, everything should be the same,

Researchers generally say that it is psilocybin, with the same spectrograph, indicating all mushroom types should produce the same experience if the same amount is taken.

The experience was different, especially when I was coming out. Usually, there are no lasting effects. This time even two hours later, I could still feel almost like a field around me that I could not shake. It was a heavy field that extended beyond the edges of my body.

I reported, "I have a lot more feeling this time. The vibration also seems to be a different, finer, or higher frequency." This is important because feeling and emotions are a big part of the psilocybin session. Usually, the vibration makes me feel like I need to go to the bathroom; therefore, I do not drink for 7 hours before my sessions. This time, I drank coffee two hours before and had no desire to use the bathroom at all.

This experience was not mystical at all. The dose, however, was exceptionally low. As it began, I listened to the beautiful music and felt that I could lean into the music and intensify it many times. I could also feel the emotion that went into the song as if I was the musician composing it.

The other odd thing in this session was that I heard songs in their sections. I could make out the words and listen to parts of the orchestra playing as if they were separated from the rest of the instruments.

However, I am only one person making this report between two different strains of mushrooms. Although this is limited information, it is much more than a scientist who has not had the experience and is looking in from the outside.

This observation of different experiences with different species of mushrooms is necessary to establish because:

- The commercialization of this medicine will be limited to laboratory-produced psilocybin only, which Drug Science chief pharmacologist David Nutt, from London College, says will cost £1500. This is the wholesale price per *dose* FOR PURE PSILOCYBIN. The industry won't allow drug trials to use natural mushrooms because it is impossible to have a standard potency. They want to synthesize it so it isn't contaminated and it is pure, so it is easier to regulate.

  To this cost, one must pay for 16 hours of pre-therapy with two therapists just to get accepted into the program, add 16 more hours of therapy with two therapists for the post-integration, plus hospital and doctors' costs).

- There is also the issue of going from taking the raw food mushroom to a synthesized drug. If the price is through the roof for insurance, it will not be covered as SSRIs (selective serotonin reuptake inhibitors) are cheap and labeled "safe and effective." The SSRI's at 1 £/pill/day. If it's 1% effective over the placebo, they can put *safe and effective* on the label. The insurance company will now pay for it, but only for the cheapest dose.

- If the mushrooms produce different experiences, the present psilocybin research is putting out false information related to the process and active ingredients.

Act 2

This experience went back to Session #1, where I felt compassion for all people suffering in the world. It also recalled Session #3, where I went through all sorts of death scenes.

This experience led me to all the people who were suffering from the COVID-19 virus. Probably I was taken there because it was on my mind. I felt the death of all these people. That day 120,000+ people had been diagnosed with the COVID-19 virus, and 1200 had died.

Feeling these events happened twice in this session, and all I could say was, "I'm sorry." I thanked them for their lives, for all the love they shared, for the things they had built, for the families they raised. I could feel the powerful experience of love that they had for the people around them.

What I perceived was the pain of the people around the dying person. Many people who die have someone at their bedside praying for a cure or more time. If you have been at the bedside of a dying person, you know that at the moment of death, there is a sudden sense of loss like "It's over. They're gone. I cannot believe it. We have lost the battle. They have died."

It was that moment of sudden realization by those who are deeply involved in that person's life that I had felt. It was one after another after another. I felt the love from the dying person for all the people that they left behind. I could also sense the memories of the dying people and what they had left behind. Thinking of the million people who had died from the virus, I could feel many good memories – all good memories of love affairs, memories of their children, travel, family. All these left behind and left for us to learn from. Here is a segment from the session tape of what I sensed:

> *It's all about memories. When you leave, you leave all of your memories. All the beautiful memories. So many ordinary people with beautiful songs they have left behind. Hundreds of thousands of memories are floating out over the land. Memories as far as the eye can see. It is like I am up on a mountain looking down over a city, and there are all these memories,*

> *beautiful memories floating around from all these people. The sun is reflecting off them. Thank you for the memories. Beautiful.*

This power of memories was evident years back when I visited the Vietnam War Memorial in Washington D.C. An outsider would just see a wall with the names of over 50,000 on it.

However, I wandered along and looked at all the cards and flowers that were left for people who had died so many years ago. One letter was from a boy who had been a young child when his father died. He wrote about how young he was and how he wished to have known his Dad, and how much he missed him. Many such letters remind us that life is about relationships, memories, and love.

Another image that came to me was related to how we start in life and then somehow pick up our beliefs along the way:

> *The reverence of life springs up. It starts with a bud springing from the ground. Before we take on the anger and hatred, we are this innocent little bud coming out of the earth, gentle and innocent. We create a story like a little girl ballet dancing or someone doing art. In the end, we look back at what we have achieved.*

Act 3

I was shown that this is part of how the universe operates. The universe is busy doing its thing based on the laws that were set up in the beginning. There is death, but there is also a universe busy creating. The universe had male or female aspects working together as a choir with men and women singing, with endless, constant motion building, building, and building. I sensed a swirling motion and action, high energy, splendor, and magnificence. It left me with this repeated sense of awe and the desire to yell Bravo!

Then came the memories of my 91-year-old mother, who was a big fan of Donald Trump. When he lost, she asked me, "What will I do now?"

In the session, this came to mind, and I realized my mother had many good memories of her own to look back on, and I have many good memories with her.

She had done more for me than her other children, and part of my integration would be to thank her, as I had failed to do this. I was sorry that I did not say, Thank you to my mother more. My family was one of those where everyone respected and loved each other, but no one showed emotion or expressed their feelings.

Session 11– Ego Death – Get Over Yourself

As I was a bit disappointed in the lack of significant events in Session #10, I decided to up the dosage to 4 grams for the Penis Envy type of mushrooms. As the rumor goes, this strain of mushrooms was created by Terence and his brother Dennis McKenna.

As with Session #10, I wanted to see if these mushrooms were different from the Golden Teacher strain or if all mushrooms are the same because they all contain psilocybin. Looking back, I would say they are different. I did not have to go to the bathroom, which was a common situation with the Teachers, and the aftereffect from these was much more potent. With the Teachers, my head was clear at the four-hour mark, and these had a hangover effect that lasted hours.

The internet is all over the map as to how powerful these mushrooms are. Some say 50% stronger; some say double. One claim said triple.

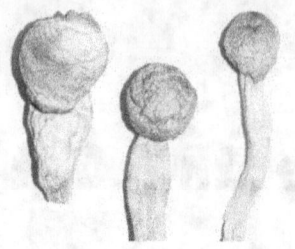

Penis Envy is one of the most **rare and sought after** Psilocybe Cubensis amongst hardcore psychonauts. Its name describes it's physical form; thick shaft and a bulbous head that doesn't quite spread wide open.

The Penis Envy strain of magic mushrooms are known to be one of the **strongest and hard hitting**. Expect deep shamanic experiences, vision quests and an intense mystical experience. **Not recommended for first time users**. This strain is special and expect a transformative experience.

I had gone for a long walk to get prepared for the trip and came back late. This caused me to start later than intended, at 7:45 pm, so the session did not end till 2:45 am.

The experience was very draining. Unlike meditation, where your mind wanders, this trip state has your mind focused on the dancing bears and the messages. There is no mind wandering. It is incredibly exhausting.

During this experience, a significant change was that during the peak part of the trip, from 1.5 hours to 4 hours, I do not remember the music, unlike the Teachers, where the music seemed to be responsible for guiding my entire trip.

What did remain the same was the critical component of *focus*. The mind appears to be floating around in the trip experience as ideas, emotions, and messages float by. As they move into awareness, I found that the witness must focus on the item. That makes it come into sharper focus. When the direction cannot be held, the object disappears and is completely lost. The process is like losing a train of thought in a discussion. Instantly, there is no recall at all of what the subject of the item was. I witnessed this many times.

I often get a backache because I am tensed up, sensing and staying in this still position, trying not to move. In this session, my mouth was parched as it was open for a prolonged period, as if I was frozen as I watched the show.

The *examining* component also appears to be critical. What you concentrate on comes into focus and can be observed. Once your focus moves, the scene disappears. Therefore, I am always focusing, which takes plenty of energy.

In fact, at about the five-hour mark, I pleaded *with the force* to let me rest. I was completely drained of energy. But *the force* behind everything just kept on going like the Energizer Bunny. So, it was up to me to break the connection. This could only be done when I took off the headset. While the music played, I was trapped on the edge of my seat, watching and simultaneously getting worn down.

Act 1

Discouraged with Session #10 and mushrooms in general, I took 4 grams of the Penis Envy, which is a lot. I was even considering stopping my psilocybin experiment because everything was so music-driven, and I did not think I was getting the noetic breakthrough that I hoped for.

I took the mushrooms in capsules this time and then meditated for about 5 minutes. I limited the time because once the plant medicine kicks in, the physical world takes a back seat, and if I am moving around, it is very disorienting.

Once under the covers, and still, I slip into the field. There is no disorientation or fear. I put on the music, headset, and blindfold and get under the covers. The wait then began.

I started at 7:45 pm, and usually, within about 20 minutes, I feel the vibration in my body; I feel like I'm floating, and if there are colors, then this is when they begin. The colors only last a few minutes, and once I pass through them, I get above the clouds where the real show begins.

Nothing seemed to be happening, so I looked at the time. I was coming up on 1.5 hours with no effects whatsoever. I had already been disappointed with the Penis Envy experience the week before, so now I felt down and out.

I laughed and thought they must have sold me your typical garden button mushrooms that you cook with a steak, and I should ask for my money back.

No word of a lie; within seconds of my thoughts, the trip started. It went from nothing to full throttle in seconds. It was almost like "they" heard my complaint and said, "You think nothing is happening? Watch this!!" They then lit the match and ignited the Saturn-V booster rocket.

I never really get colors and shapes, but this time I got them big time. It was not fun. I only remember a tiny bit. Here is what I said in the recording. I entered the realm with the same song that I had heard during my past trips. The audio confirms this was only seconds after I looked at the clock:

Same psychedelic colors, yellow, green, vibration in my higher back, vibration when I speak, swirling colors, same yellow psychedelic colors, small dots in the colors, the first time I have seen light blue.

Intense vibration. Choking. Gold, sparkly (gold is a first). Intense closeness. Pressure, pain in the left side of my chest, extreme vibration, pain above my heart. Different colors this time, goldish pink, sparkling, twinkling, light on the left-hand side. Streaks of light, sparkly, yellow with purple, like a snowflake. A dark light, if that makes sense. Right above me, vibration, a colored snowflake structure looking down at me, intense pressure on my chest. Intense, fierce, beautiful light colors.

The pressure on the left side of my chest. Very immediate sensation, slowly swirling to the right. It is mixing with the music. Intense, intense pressure on the left side, above my heart. Color streaking up. Some pain in my left chest, vibration, color. Now brightness. Colors are coming in these weird psychedelic outlines. The vibration is now down my left side.

Again, if I concentrate on the color, it intensifies. These colors are very, very close to me, yellow-brown, intense vibration. They are close but in the darkness. The outline gives the impression of everything being lit up...

Often, while in the experience, it starts with some dark presence that slowly moves across my body about 1 inch above me. The sense is that this "thing" is observing me and testing my panic reaction. I stay very still as it moves over, and then it just goes away as if I passed the test.

The same thing happened this time, but it was followed by these colored wire structures that were moving around me and coming close in. It was very annoying. One form looked like a one-foot-long mechanical insect made of colored links like a bicycle chain. Here is that section of the tape:

Hard to relax. I feel like a very old man. (hard time finding the tape recorder) This is very disorienting. I can see a very sort of colorful structure, getting closer, hard to describe. Is it made of little pieces of a chain? Not touching. Green, blue-purple. Intense pressure and vibration on my chest. The things are getting closer, closer, really close. The music is slowing down. Almost like this thing is right below me. 'Hello.' (I am now talking to it) 'Hello. How are you doing? Come on.' So, I am trying to describe this. Intense Pressure. I am looking at the backside. It is made of, what is this? Let's go to something half decent. What is this nonsense? It is like I have to feed my hallucination. It is entirely silent. Everything has stopped except for the vibration. So, everything has stopped.

Holy cow!! A commercial (on Spotify) has come on now. It is kind of weird. It is like this is very vibratory. Okay. It still seems to be there. I tried to tell it to go away. To take ownership of it. It is very, very light. Vibratory sensation. Hmmm. Okay, so weird. It is like they are bending the vision of something. Okay, they are doing this vision thing. It is like an utterly physical type of experience. So, I have this - they are messing with it, totally messing with reality.

The whole episode was getting me very distressed, and I thought, "I am not going to put up with this." I started to panic a bit, thinking I may have overdone the dose, and would now spend eternity with these silent, slow-moving things all around me.

Thinking back on what I had read do under this circumstance, someone said that you could tell the "things" to leave. So, I said, "This is my experience, and I need you to leave RIGHT NOW." Nothing happened. They were still around me and very close. The silence and slow movement were extremely tense. I tried it again. Nothing. Then I panicked:

Okay, it's bizarre. Multi-colored, and the vibration is like this swirling pattern. So, if I make it go away – If I say 'GO AWAY. GO AWAY.' (nothing happens) No. It is going along with the music. It wouldn't say this is a positive experience. It has lit up, and I have to try and remember that I am a human being. It is doing this weird thing. It is all a multi-colored structure. There is something that I would say, it is weird. I can't really stop it, so it is bizarre, it doesn't matter what they are playing. Wow, this is not a positive experience. There are these lines that are vibrating. It's in color. It's lit, and there are these lines that are vibrating. They are sending electricity down these various colored lines. Wow. Why would I see this? This is insane. So, they control the color, but they don't control the music. They control the vibration. What is going on? If you tell them 'stop it stop it!!' Would they stop? No. This kind of throws me for a loop. This is like a very visual negative experience, and there is nothing I can do to stop it.

That led to me doing the correct thing. I gave up and let go and decided that this could continue for 4 hours, or maybe forever. Almost instantaneously, I moved back and watched them - now much further away from my body. My panic and fear left once I surrendered and owned the fact that I had done the high dose. I was now just an observer, and I broke into the field for the experience:

> *Trust, let go and be open. So, let's try letting go. Okay. It becomes a lot less. It becomes a positive experience when you let go—(a long pause). Okay (laughs), I keep forgetting I am on tape. This is messing with my reality. (laughs) I like to know that you are here. (laughs again) (Pause then more laughter) They are showing it to me again. (laughs) Ahhh*
>
> *What's the universe? Up we go. That you are – (laughs) – now I am through to the other side I forget that I am recording. (long pause) Holy shit! (laughs) You have no idea. Ahh. Ahhh. Ahhhh (laughs) You have not got a clue. I saw it. Unbelievable! (laughs) Oh my God. I can't explain. It is almost like I didn't (trails off), Almost like I was shown. I keep thinking about reality. (laughs) Holy shit. Beyond belief. The ah, If you think you know what's going on, good luck! The beauty they show it to me. You go out of time and space. Thank you. (Laughter) Unbelievable. Ohh. They are showing me how it works. There is emotion. I knew that already. The vibration emotion. BRAVO! Unbelievable. (whispering) You haven't got a clue, folks. They showed me. I saw it for, again, they showed me. I have been shown how it works. (Laughs) They showed me. The vibration (inaudible)Love. (Long pause) They showed me how reality works. I am so honored.*

So, what did I see? There were long periods where I watched. I was laughing through the whole thing and repeated statements like "Unbelievable," "Holy shit," "People have no clue," "Thank you," "They are showing me." This went on for at least 30 minutes. I, however, have no clue what I saw. This corresponded with the other two sessions where I encountered this force and believed I was shown something.

Yet, there was not much on the audio where I described what I was seeing. A possible answer came from the recording I made during the session. I heard myself say, "They make you forget it as soon as you see it," and "You forget it as soon as you see it – that's the deal."

Here are some things that I said that might hint at what I was seeing from a female force. It should be pointed out that I laughed through this whole thing like it was the funniest thing I had ever seen. "Life is an illusion." "How it came- how it does it." "Will take a while to integrate." "Showed me the positive and negative mixed with sensory." "It was all made up." "They make me question my whole life as to what happened." "They go after all that I know to be true, devastating; my whole life was made up." "Reality was all made up, and they let me see it." (I said this more than four dozen times.) "It's not as important as I thought it was." "I am getting the absolute sense of it." "They want people to know it's all made up." "The universe made it all up." "They are running it." I said, "To sense it, to know, to feel it. I don't know what to think." "As serious as you thought about your politics, and your life, your love, and your hate, the Universe just made it up." "The hate... we thought we were so smart and had it all figured out, but it was all made up, and now it is showing off" (laughing.) "The whole idea of people and a planet. They made it up." "They are showing me the idea of countries and planets and people, ego, me and you. Just made it up."

Act 2

As 95% of my trips' memories have disappeared into thin air, the key thing I remember was talking to what I call *the force*. This is how I would characterize *the force*. I was busy thinking about describing 'it' as the experience was happening. This is at least the third encounter I have had with this force.

- I could sense but not see *the force*.
- I know it. I know what it is. It does not have to tell me.
- It is alive.
- It <u>appears</u> to be swirling counterclockwise. This is just a sense.
- It appears to be the thing that is behind creation.
- It is a verb. I got this in my 2017 noetic experience as well. There are only verbs. Everything is part of *the force*, and it is alive. There are NO NOUNS. Our left brain is trying to turn everything into a world of separation, where everything is just an object in a random, meaningless universe.
- It again appeared to come across as female energy. It can also come across as male, but that may be confused with seeing *the force* as this powerful influence behind creation that leaves one with the feeling of magnificence and awe, like some powerful king.

- It has unlimited energy. It just keeps creating at full speed. It does not rest. It drained my energy in a couple of hours.
- It is entirely neutral. It sets all laws in place, and everything that is happening is a result of that. It is not good or bad. Everything is perfect. We attach meanings to things.
- *The force* is very blunt with the messages. It does not beat around the bush. In a way, that is what I wanted, so it could be that this is all just a reflection of myself. At times I have thought, "how could you say that to me?" Until I thought about it and then realized that *the force* was right on the mark. (An example of this bluntness would be Mother Ayahuasca talking to Dennis McKenna, where he was told, "You monkeys just think you are in charge.")
- I could communicate with this force. The music was a key component of communication. It was almost like the message I received from Chris Bledsoe that, "the message is in the music." The messages were *sensed*, which is hard to explain unless you have experienced this.
- It has a sense of humor, or it is pretending to, as that breaks down my defenses.
- Again, I got the sense that it was showing off. I have a theory about it. When you sense it, it seems powerful, magnificent, and awe-inspiring. As with everything else in this non-local field, it intensifies five or ten

times when you focus on something. Therefore, when I focus on *the force*, it strengthens, making it look like it is showing off. This happened many times. I would be laughing and saying, "Yeah, you go, girl." When you focus on *the force*, it is breathtaking, extremely emotional, and must be where the word AWE comes from.

- It leaves you with the sense that you are being shown something of utmost importance. It left me feeling like I was the luckiest person in the world, and I was honored that I would be shown this. I kept saying, Thank you. I felt like a Messiah and that I should go out and create a new religion. I can now see how religious movements get going. An encounter with *the force* is a compelling and moving experience.

- *The force* always leaves you with a sense of reverence.

Act 3

Once again, *the force* gave me an essential message. At one point, the message was "Grant. It is time to get over yourself. I just made you up." I had to run this message a couple of times and got a revelation.

I said, "You made me up?"

The reply came, "Yup, and everything else."

The concept has been around for a long time that the universe was just an idea in the creator's mind. That is generally accepted. When I was told that I was a character that *the force* had made up and put on a stage, it was still shocking. It felt like the ultimate putdown. I went from ego Grant to something that was made up.

This feeling is described as part of a mystical state's characteristics, sometimes called the diminished self. There is "an overwhelming sense of awe at 'your' (now non-existent) insignificance in comparison to the vastness of existence."

So, now I was being told that everything was all made up. *The force* decided to make up a story that involved a universe, the big bang, and everything else. It threw in some galaxies and stars with planets. The humans were an idea as well, and then *the force* decided to make them different colors for learning purposes and *the force's* entertainment. The concept of God, life after death, and Donald Trump are real but just made up of consciousness *the force*.

Reality is real to those in the play, but our reality is essentially just a thought. We come to believe we are the characters on the stage, but it is all made up. The goal in life is to remember who we are. We are not the actor on the stage, nor are we the thoughts in our heads. We are the observers of the play.

I laughed and continued to chuckle until *the force* showed me how it had been done. At one point, I recall that I was creating it as well. When it became apparent to me this play scenario had happened and that I was just a creation in *the force's* mind, the only analogy that I can think of is that my foot slipped. I grabbed for something to hang on to, and there was nothing there.

It was like slipping and grabbing and realizing you have fallen off of the Empire State building. There was a sudden massive sense of loss. It was over. All that I thought was real was gone. It was a scary feeling beyond words.

It was the ultimate ego death. My life and how I see reality will never be the same. The collapse of the ego as an idea is not that threatening. But when it happens in the nonlocal field as a real event, it can be earth-shattering.

According to the New York Times, this correct understanding of the "I" made Eckhart Tolle "the most popular spiritual author in the United States" in 2008.

I couldn't live with myself any longer. A question arose without an answer: "Who is the 'I' that cannot live with the self?" "What is the self?" I felt drawn into a void! I didn't know it, but what had happened was my mind-made *self*, with its heaviness, its problems, that lives between the unsatisfying past and the fearful future, had collapsed. It dissolved. The next morning, I woke up, and everything was so peaceful. The peace was there because there was no *self*. Just a sense of presence or "beingness," just observing and watching.

Act 4

Once again, during the finale of the trip, I looked back on my life and thought that it had been a good life. I also realized that I had to clear up my relationship with my mother and others. This job was not yet complete.

This whole realization was inspired by Wolfgang Mozart "Klarinettenkonzert A-Dur, K. 622: Adagio (Jenseits von Africa): 11. Adagio," as it was the session before this one when it played.

Act 5

In the end, I destroyed the recording of this session as it was so repetitive. I also resolved to do the next session without music and keep my commentary down to ten minutes to gather the main ideas that came up.

The essence of the message in Session #11 was a reminder of the old Eastern concept that we are not the bodies we live in. We give substance to the clay that makes us up, and when it rains, the clay melts away back to the Earth. We forget that we are not the object we think we are. We are just the observers of our bodies and the things around us.

Some believe in the Hindu concept of Maya, which was the magic power with which a god can make human beings believe that this world is real when, in fact, it is an illusion.

The Isha Upanishad states, "the Brahman, forms everything that is living or non-living ... the wise man knows that all beings are identical with his self, and his self is the self of all beings."

The fact that we are not the individuals we think we are was summed up by physicist, Nobel Laureate, Erwin Schrödinger:

In itself, the insight is not new. The earliest records, to my knowledge, date back some 2500 years or more... the recognition ATMAN = BRAHMAN (the personal self-equals the omnipresent, all-comprehending eternal self) was in Indian thought considered, far from being blasphemous, to represent the quintessence of deepest insight into the happenings of the world.

Session 12 – Gotcha

I had run into *the force* three times by this point. Tonight, I would meet it again, and this encounter would have the drama of the most dynamic Broadway musical. The Universe loves drama, and that is how it delivers its messages so that the experiencer will never forget. The encounter I was about to have would rival any I had ever read. And this is because it happened to me and came with the excitement, emotion, vibration, and reverence that you cannot get from a dull lecture on mystical experiences.

I wrote up this session in a manuscript but was not considering publishing it. It appeared that I had not gotten anything that was independent and convincing in my attempt to break through into a higher realm.

I decided to continue to use the powerful mushrooms but wanted to drop the dosage to 3 grams. This was done because the 4 grams I had consumed the week before had created an audio recording that started well but ended up being real laughter with the constant repetition of the idea that reality is Maya – illusion.

Feeling that things had not gone deep enough, I decided to do the session without music and in a state of meditation. Johns Hopkins University did an experiment where long-term meditators consumed high-dose psilocybin with excellent results.

My mediation was totally set up. I would sit on the bed against the wall and set up pillows to support my knees for what would be 4 hours in the lotus position.

The drama started right from the opening minutes. The Muse device that would monitor my brainwaves to stay in the zone was low on power. Therefore, I set up my second computer on the bed to charge the Muse while going into the field.

I also had the audio recorder but was determined to speak for no more than 10 minutes only when something big happened.

After taking the medicine, everything started to go south. It was impossible to wear a blindfold and use the Muse simultaneously because both required using my ears. I would worry about that later.

Starting, I did a compassion meditation, a gratitude one, and an awareness one. I repeated these three several times. The vibration was taking over my body. It got more and more intense. So far, so good.

What followed was something that might be a pattern in the psilocybin experience. There was some sort of challenging event that leads to an elevated grand vision of the other side. In four of the 12 sessions I had completed, something came very close to my body.

The first two gave the impression of a large black object moving to slowly only an inch over me on the bed. It caused some concern, so I lay still, and it seemed to end. In Session #11, the objects were visible and seemed intent on unnerving me. In Session #12, I would experience almost a full-on attack.

A week after this, I wondered if it was some kind of paranormal pattern. Maybe something to kill the ego before showing higher-level concepts? There are examples inside Ufology that are similar:

- In the abduction or contact experience, a being appears in the experiencer's bedroom and wakes the person up. Immediately, one is engaged with a being in their bedroom looking at them. This has to be the most frightening thing that one can imagine. Why would beings do such a thing? It appears to be some sort of process that causes dissociation, which I pointed out in my book, *Contact Modalities: The Keys to the Universe*. This scenario could be a means for getting a person into the non-local field.

- In UFO military sightings, there is often a situation where the sightings, like my psilocybin experiences, involve an object coming very close. An example is of an incident where jets on the nuclear aircraft carrier, USS Theodore Roosevelt, saw what looked like small spheres inside of cubes that flew within inches of the aircraft during multiple flybys. The fear the pilots must have felt is identical to the ego death I experienced when I felt the object's presence near my bed and was scared to death; clearly, the phenomenon runs the show. Why would the UFOs do this except to cause some sort of reaction of helplessness?

- In another case, within the last 12 months, a large triangular object came up out of the water near a submarine, which caused total panic. The UFO allowed an F-18 in the air to catch the whole thing on record.
- In the 1970s, a UFO circled a nuclear missile test site out of Vandenburg AFB and disabled the rocket over the Pacific as the downrange cameras filmed the entire incident.

This same drama occurred to me in Session #12, but it was much more dramatic than past events. It became a *real* drama. I sensed some colors and wavy things floating around. Suddenly, I heard a high-pitched grating sound. I had never heard that sound before but wondered if that was because there was no music to drown it out. A small colored pinpoint of light flew by me at a very high speed and was very close to me. It had an orbit like a planet, and I was in the middle.

Then there was another light and another. Each was emitting this terrible sound. I ignored these fast-moving objects, but they did not stop. It got worse. I repeated the mantra, "Trust, let go, be open." Nothing happened. It was getting ugly, and the panic was setting in as I tried to control it. I concentrated closely on my breath, and it got worse.

I started to wonder how anyone could do a session without the music. Did everyone without music have to put up with what was quickly becoming hell for me? There was no exit door, and I was stuck. Everything I tried made it worse. I was now in a living hell, and panic broke out.

The situation made me irate, and I thought, "I am so glad I decided not to put out the book because it would be pulled if this was written. If one person reads the book and ends up in this hell, it would be my fault. After 11 good sessions, how could this one go so bad?

As my anger grew, so did the bombardment of these high-pitched lights that were racing around me. How could some mushroom, or the Universe for that matter, be so evil to create this kind of situation? I had tried everything, but the situation continued to get worse. The last thing I tried was to lower my head to tolerate better what was happening.

The session had just started, and it became evident that this would be my experience for the next few hours. My worldview was shattered because I had long preached that trips could be controlled if you knew what you were doing. I had been wrong. There was evil in the world, and I was now living with it for the next four hours or possibly for eternity.

Why had this scenario never happened when I was listening to music? It appeared this might be my only hope to survive what was happening. It was time to get in the lifeboat. The planned session was over as I was heading for the covers and the music. It was all that was left to do.

I disassembled my meditation set-up in the dark, rearranging pillows and finding my playlist. Everything was so much harder to do as my left brain had been disabled. I went to take my computer off sleep mode but could not figure out how to turn it on. Now frustration was also setting in.

Finally, I got my computer working and managed to find Spotify. I struggled to click on the Johns Hopkins playlist and ended up clicking on another playlist. (This would turn out to be a good thing). The music was wrong, and I wondered if I should leave it to play. My audio recorder was lost. To hell with it. I went to get under my covers but couldn't figure out how to pull them back. After many frustrating attempts, I realized the computer was still on the bed, holding the covers down. It occurred to me to just throw it on the floor, but I nicely moved it to the desk once I calmed down a bit. All this was done in complete darkness.

Act 1

Under the covers, I went with the wrong music playing. Within seconds I was in my familiar bubble. I am not sure whether those annoying lights were still attacking me. I don't recall thinking about them once I was lying down with the music and blindfold on.

Within what appeared to be seconds, my awareness started to move forward. If it were my physical body, it would have been five feet ahead of me. If it was my mind awareness, the movement was five inches. There was a corner, and my attention made a right turn at the corner. Now, I could feel what was down from the corner.

I was facing *the force,* Universe, or whatever name you want to give it. There was an immediate recognition and the usual and utter sense of reverence. It was right there.

A direct message was issued from *the force.* It said "Gotcha!" and then started to laugh. I began to laugh. Then I knew why the adverse event happened. I thought back to many sessions before where I was referenced as the *ignorant ego* who would be smart and figure it all out. It had happened again.

"I" had been frustrated at the process in the sessions, and "I" had taken things into my own hands. "I" would figure out how to get into the field. "I" would use mediation and come in from the back door where *the force* wouldn't see "me." "I" had plans to walk downstairs to deepen the trance mentally. "I" had it all figured out. In "my" frustration for results, "I" had taken control of the situation.

The same thing had happened the session before, and I had not picked up on the message again. Therefore, this time the message was delivered with a bit more drama. The hellish part of the experience greeted "me" and drove me into submission. It turned me into a cowering little boy hiding in my bed.

As soon as "I" surrendered, "I" was free, and it was over. The message was, "Surrender is the only rule. Believe me, surrender is the only rule." That is how I got it. Like the session before, my ego was crushed; and I laughed *when the force* pointed out the rules again.

It was as if I was in Hawaii in mid-January, and there had been a lot of turbulence on the flight in. According to a bad trip survey conducted at Johns Hopkins, this flip from bad to good is not that uncommon. They reported the following:

> *Thirty-four percent of participants said the 'bad trip' was among the top five most personally meaningful experiences of their life, and 31 percent said it was among the top five most spiritually significant. And 76 percent said their bad trip had resulted in an improved sense of personal well-being or life satisfaction. Forty-six percent said they would be willing to experience the lousy trip all over again.[18]*

Some might consider the Universe to be cruel and see that this was a dirty trick to play. My take from my experiences is that the Universe is just and sometimes comes across as cruel when we don't get fed candy all the time like we think we deserve.

A similar incident occurred when Dr. Michael Newton was regressing a client. Dr. Newton created the *Life Between Life* research work after regressing 7,000 clients and taking them into the spirit world between lives.

Newton's story was that of a man who had lived a past life as a fire and brimstone preacher. As Newton led the man to die and go into the spirit world, he suddenly cried out that he was face to face with Satan.

Newton asked him how he knew it was Satan and what did Satan look like? The man was devastated, saying he knew that he was in hell. He described Satan's leathery skin, which led to Newton asking what the beast was wearing. The man responded but reported that there was nobody below the waist.

Newton told the man he was not in hell, but the man would not listen. Newton said that this did not make sense and asked the man to "Take a closer look. Who is it really?"

The man got quiet as he looked and then declared that his spirit guide was posing as Satan. The lesson was to get the man a taste of the fire and brimstone he was spouting to his congregation. He said that his spirit guide often used masks to teach him lessons. The man was satisfied that he had it coming. The message was delivered.

That may be one of the most important things to realize about the psychedelic experience. In the physical world, we can use talk therapy to convince people to change their habits. We know, for a fact, that in most cases, it is ineffective. One figure claims that talk therapy for alcohol use disorder is 2% effective. That compares to a Johns Hopkins meta-analysis of randomized studies using lysergic acid diethylamide (LSD) for alcohol use disorder (AUD) which showed 83% no longer met AUD criteria so were cured.[19]

Act 2

Now that I was in the field. I was shown something about the Universe but then immediately forgot it. I got the message that bringing the information back was not allowed. I did leave the experience with a sense of awe at the complexity of how life operates.

This time I was shown something in which one second of the event remained with me. I am not sure if that was an error or allowed me to remember what I saw. The maybe two seconds I saw had to do with the plasticity of the higher realms. This has been reported by lucid dreamers, psychonauts, and UFO experiencers.

I saw part of a half-visible body, and the movement I saw was a right arm moving inward towards the body. The whole image was smeared as if the arms were in all the positions at the same time. This gave the impression of a photo on a rubber surface that is then stretched. Simultaneously, every vertical piece of the stretched image was independent, and parts were able to move up and down.

Some might say this is a hallucination, but it had a sense that I was being shown a principle of the plasticity of reality and that it was only a small part of the larger piece, which I forgot right as it happened.

Act 3

For many years, I have read about the experience of being in a field of unconditional love. If I could achieve a lucid dream, it would be the first thing I would ask for. This phenomenon is probably most reported in near-death-experiences when the person encounters Jesus, God, or the light at the end of the tunnel.

In this session, I was able to experience it. My memory is clear, and the experience appeared to continue for an extended period. Then the experience unfolded.

Earlier in the day, I was part of a conversation with Deb Frueh, a tarot card reader in Illinois, who runs a yearly metaphysical gathering for practitioners. She was talking about the death of her son, who had struggled in life.

At some point during my experience that night, I felt the unconditional love that the Universe has for everyone. I sensed being told that love could be equated to the love a mother has for her child.

The message is that a person could be the lowest creature to walk the Earth, yet their mother would still love them. That is the love the universe has for everyone, no matter what they have done or not done in life.

The next thing that I recall was a life review. It consisted of confronting *the force* and placing all my mistakes and sins in front of it. I walked in feeling that this was judgment day. I put all my baggage in front of *the force* and bowed my head in regret. It was all exposed.

The force looked down on all I had presented. At that moment, I could feel an arm around my shoulder and heard the words. "It's okay, Grant. It's okay." My take was that the universe could have cared less what I had exposed. It was only interested in comforting me with unconditional forgiveness.

It was at this moment that I found myself in this field of unconditional love and acceptance. As in many experiences I have had with the field, I felt gratitude and a feeling of being deeply loved and appreciated. I really can't add anything to the many accounts similar to this that can be found on the internet.

Act 4

Another feeling that I experienced was the state of absolute bliss. I have had this before, as have probably millions who have had mystical experiences. In this state, I reached for words knowing that it would be impossible but that I would attempt to write about it.

The only words that come to mind were vibration and emotion. Most mystical experiences have a vital emotional component in them, which is extremely hard to translate because bliss does not often happen in daily life. The closest thing I can associate with this feeling is being in a huge crowd when a standing ovation occurs, and the emotion of the group swells and can be experienced by all.

Bach programmed it as the finale to a ten-movement liturgical work celebrating the miraculous pregnancies of Mary and Elizabeth from the Gospel of Luke, and God's subversion of the world order through the birth of Christ. "The wondrous hand of the exalted Almighty is active in the mysteries of the earth!" the work proclaims.

Session 13

This is the chapter I never intended to write. After the negative experience of Chapter 12 and feeling that I had gotten the answers that I was seeking, it was time to move on to other topics for study.

Still, I had about 5 grams of the high potency mushrooms left and three grams that were already cut up and needed to be used. It was time to try again.

Act 1

Because of a very hellish experience in the previous session and a less harrowing experience the time before that, I was very hesitant going into the experience. The brand of mushrooms I was using provided all the "bad trips" I had undergone. This proved to me that it wasn't just the psilocybin in the mushroom. The species of mushroom used seemed to provide different experiences.

As my difficult Session #12 had begun in silence while trying to meditate, I decided to go back to the music. When I finally gave in and put on the playlist, everything shifted and got better. I, therefore, made sure to start and finish with the music.

Like the previous two sessions with the Penis Envy mushrooms, there was a brief moment when the "bad trip" started again. I quickly stopped it, which led me to understand further why the "bad" was happening.

The event occurred while I was closing in on the middle of the trip. A song had ended, and there was a pause before the next musical piece. The time during the break was very long. I wondered why this was happening and thought that the music had stopped because there was no computer activity. That would mean that I would have to get up and restart the program.

While waiting, I sensed that the silence had a texture to it, an actual essence. This was not unusual. I had felt this before. Then came what was a sound of cracking as water quickly freezes.

What I observed was that I was looking into a square box. Within two seconds, the cracking sound became sharp, like ice shards forming from all the walls of the container extending into the middle. What I saw were faces that looked like they were straight out of a horror movie starting to form in the ice shards.

I said, "This is happening," and I quickly removed the blindfold and sat up. The image was gone, and the playlist went to commercial. After calming down, I put on the blindfold again, laid down, and was back in the beautiful bubble of the experience once again.

Thinking about this, I hypothesized that the silence had been the problem as silence was a big part of the session 12 bad trip segment. When the music is on, it guides your mind through reflective, sad, happy, and upbeat songs. When silence is there, the brain gets to fill in the void.

The long pause caused the fear to enter. As soon as the pause was too long, I sensed something was wrong. Why was it so long, and why do I hear this silence? I was not surprised at the jagged ice and faces appearing. It fit the mood of my mind at that moment. That is why I quickly removed the blindfold and moved to the computer to solve the silence. It had just gone to a commercial, and I immediately felt better.

As Nobel Laureate John Wheeler stated, "It's a participatory universe."

Act 2 – The Colors and Shapes

The Penis Envy mushrooms have great mystical powers from my experience, but they produce some turbulence getting to altitude. To get to a breakthrough state, you must go through the clouds to get to the appropriate altitude.

With this strain, people can expect to see the colored geometrical shapes as the trip begins. These colors and shapes only last for the first 15 minutes or so once the effects of the psilocybin take hold.

If one reads the psychedelic literature, one gets the idea that this *is* the experience. It is not, at least in my own 13 trips. It often doesn't happen at all, and if it does, it is near the beginning, almost like going through psychedelic clouds to get to the higher state where the experience happens.

This idea is essential for negating the materialistic concept of everything being caused by brain chemistry where it "generates geometric visual hallucinations that are closely related to those used to process edges, contours, surfaces, and textures."

If the psilocybin caused the colored shapes, they would continue throughout the entire experience, which they don't. If the chemicals were causing the shapes, they also should last throughout the experience, as the chemical is logged onto the serotonin receptor in the brain called 5-HT2A, where psilocin (the active metabolite of psilocybin) binds to cause the psychedelic experience[20], not just at the beginning of the experience, but for the entire trip.

I had a bad experience in Chapter 12 in that the shapes were very annoying. Therefore, when they appeared this time, I was cautious to stay calm, accept what was happening, and realize that it would only go on for a few minutes.

The shapes this time were different than the orbiting objects that I experienced in Session #12, the bicycle chain qualities I saw in Session #11, and the wispy, fluorescent outlines in a few of my earlier experiences. These temporary manifestations again negate the chemical explanation. If it was a simple 5-HT2A psilocybin reaction, it should be the same every time and not just occur near the beginning of the trip.

When I saw the shapes this time, they immediately reminded me of the shapes of lines that were reported on a triangular UFO that had been in one of my recent YouTube panels on Triangle-UFO Sightings. Could I be transposing those shapes into my experience?

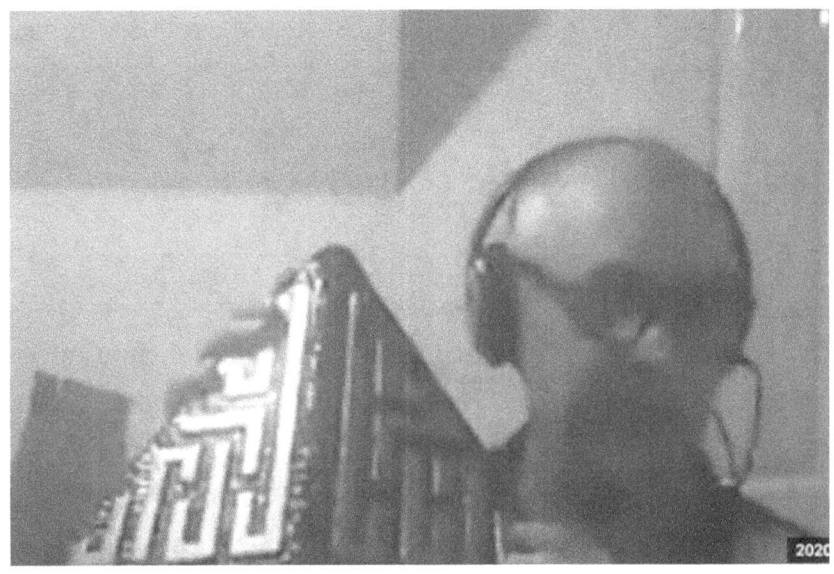

The patterns looked the same, but they were relatively far away. They extended over the entire field of vision. The inside of the shapes was made up of a row of black dots. Like all of the other colors and shapes I saw, the objects' actual formation only came into focus when I concentrated on them. By not paying attention, I could almost make them disappear.

By looking closer, I would see that the shapes were appearing on a light yellow background and consisted of the black channel lines with the black dots in between. The yellow background was also a very dim white.

Shapes appeared a couple more times before they went away, but the forms were not the same. I also saw other channels with orange fluorescent lines with black dots in the track on a black background.

I have no idea what the patterns are and why they appear at the beginning of about 50% of my sessions.

Act 3- The Noetic Experience

A few days before this trip, I was interviewed on a radio show with researcher and writer Lee Spiegel. We were talking about my 2012 and 2017 noetic experiences. Lee asked me how it feels getting the information and if I ever hear a voice.

I told him that I heard no voice. I seem only to sense things, and the information appears to be real knowledge instead of a good idea. It was as if I was talking to God and being given actual knowledge. It is challenging to describe to someone who has not ever had a noetic experience.

The noetic idea must have been an intention I took with me into the trip because during the session, I was given two answers to my noetic experiences that would help me to explain them to an outsider with no experience or to a rational, skeptical conscious mind. Here are the two explanations that came from wherever – my higher self, God, aliens, the akashic field, or whatever source we might want to attribute the knowledge to:

1) The simple explanation: Like Jesus and the Bible, the psilocybin experience seems to be more easily explained by parables and analogies. The analogy I'll use is where someone asks you a question, and immediately a reply pops into your head. "Who was your first boyfriend or girlfriend?" Right away, a name will pop into your head. That is how noetic information appears in the mind. There is no one waving a sign at you. There is no voice yelling at you. It just pops into your head. Now the skeptic on the outside will ask, "Where did the noetic name come from?" The answer is, "What difference does it make?"

   Then the skeptic will say, "How do you know that the name that came into your head is accurate?" The answer is, "Go to hell. I just know." There is a certainty about the answer, and the same type of certainty comes with noetic ideas.

2) The second explanation was more neurological. Again, the information came like the name of my first girlfriend – quickly and with certainty. It had the sense of actual knowledge because as the concept was being shown, I thought, "Oh, so that is how it works. That makes total sense."

   What I was shown was the model of a brain that is on psilocybin. The default mode network

(DMN)[21] in the brain that guides our daily lives and thoughts goes offline (when on psilocybin), as shown in fMRI research financed by the Beckley Foundation at London College. Simultaneously, the two sides of the brain start to work as one, and parts of the brain that don't normally communicate start talking to each other.

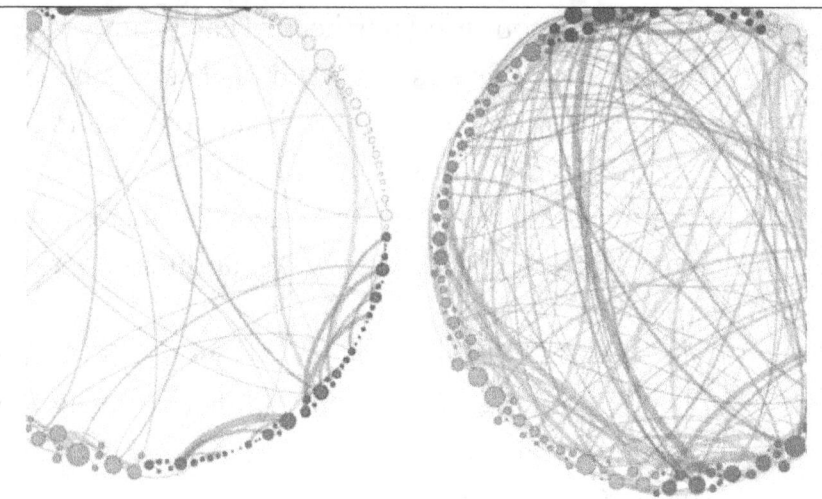

Left, the stable brain activity in a normal brain. Right, under the influence of psilocybin, diverse brain regions not normally in communication become strongly linked.

This new brain talk provides new insights into problems. This makes sense as a whole different part of the brain is now working on the issue.

I recalled two quotes that I had used often to connect them to this experience.

"We can't solve problems by using the same kind of thinking we used when we created them," and "a new type of thinking is essential if mankind is to survive and move toward higher levels."

-Albert Einstein

What happens in ordinary, daily thinking is that the DMN is online and is doing nothing more than shuffling around what was described to me through my experience as "wrong blocks."

We now have fewer *wrong blocks* than in the past, but as my 2017 noetic experience indicated, "not only do you have it wrong, it is exactly the opposite of what you think it is." The *wrong blocks* used to include erroneous beliefs that humanity had, such as the world is flat, 5,000 stars are in existence, stars are not suns, there are no other galaxies, and the sun revolves around Earth. You can rearrange those wrong blocks in any pattern till Jesus walks down 5th avenue, and you will never get the right answers. As William James pointed out, we think we are thinking, but we are just rearranging prejudices and wrong blocks.

In modern science, we continue to believe we have it all figured out, but we possibly still have many wrong blocks. This is the ego talking, assuring us that we have it figured out. In my 2017 noetic experience, however, it was pointed out that this is not true. I was shown ideas like a) Everything is made of consciousness, not nuts and bolts. b) We are living multiple lives as opposed to one life. c) The universe is built with a definite pattern and not random events. d) Everything is connected as one, and there is no separation. e) Science describes their beliefs, assuming that they used the right blocks to explain their theories. f) People think they know something when they are just believing.

We take our present wrong blocks and use the DMN to rearrange them in various patterns, leading to dead ends because the essential information is incorrect. We are trying to solve the problem using the same wrong blocks used to create the problem.

In the psilocybin experience, new wiring patterns are formed in the brain, and then new blocks can be pulled in by the new insights that the new brain pattern can access.

More importantly, the information that is being accessed is noetic. It brings with it not old prejudices but what William James called:

> *...insight into depths of truth unplumbed by the discursive intellect. They are illuminations, revelations, full of significance and importance, all inarticulate though they remain, and as a rule, they carry with them a curious sense of authority for after-time.*

Act 4 -The Life Review

I picked up some messages that seemed to come to me while listening to the music. Some felt very firm as if coming from a universe that is all-loving but no-nonsense. These are messages that even people close to me and this story may have a problem accepting. However, my impression is that the universe is neutral when changing the rules it has set up.

During one of the reflective songs, I picked up that I had to deal with something connected to my mother.

While listening to this music, I found that I was looking back at all the low parts of my life. As memories unfold, the emotions are exposed, and you can deal with them. Now they do not seem so bad. This is similar to talk therapy, where you can come to terms with issues and sort them out, so they aren't as traumatic anymore. The bizarre thing about it was that the visual review was occurring behind a shopping mall about one mile south of where I lived.

This may be how depression and PTSD can be altered and healed in the psilocybin state because there is no judgment. You are ok. It is ok. Is what the teaching offers. In the conscious world, they are more challenging to solve with either talk therapy or anti-depressant drugs. There are adverse side effects here. And rarely do we encounter the unconditional love from the universe. For myself, when the somewhat negative experiences were brought forward, they were don't so with no judgment. And with respect. It was ok to forgive myself. All was not as bad as I was afraid it would be. The feeling I was getting from whoever was rolling out the events was that "this was not as bad as you thought."

The one event that did come with a lecture was the memory of a stock deal that cost me hundreds of thousands of dollars. In this event, I was being told, "You wanted to play the game of being rich even though you preached against it. You knew that it was easier for a camel to get through the key of a needle than for a rich man to enter the kingdom of Heaven, and yet you still played. You said one thing and quietly played the get rich behind the scenes as if no one would know."

It continued, "A capitalist who had better inside information than you took your money, which was the game you chose to play. You didn't want the cash down deep, so quit with regret."

When the song was over, the regret was over, and everything was alright.

Act 5- The Love Experience

At one point, I was enveloped by the feeling of unconditional love. This is not uncommon. It was incredible, and I tried to take note of exactly how it felt. The words that I would come to find are vibration, love, comfortable, and all-encompassing. It was a place a person would never want to leave. In the end, it was probably ineffable.

While absorbing and enjoying it, I felt that I was to share this feeling with others. It was not that I was to love others, but instead, I shared the same total and unconditional love that I was feeling at that moment with both my friends and enemies.

Act 6

This was the most memorable and dramatic part of the session. It centered around two songs, which made such an impression on me, I just had to get up in 3D reality and check the playlist to see which songs they were.

Going to my computer during a session is something that I have rarely done. Usually, at the end of the session, I could not remember any single song playing the entire trip.

The other incident that was strange was that I could move in and out of the bubble with ease. When using the Golden Teacher mushrooms, I found that if I got up to restart the music or go to the bathroom, I would be very unstable, confused, and think of only one thing – getting back under the covers and back into the experience.

This time, I felt completely normal when I was up and looking into the songs, except that it was harder to do computer tasks. Then when I put the blindfold on and got under the covers, I was right back in the experience within seconds. I went in and out many times and had no problem (or at least that is what I thought). With the Golden Teacher, I found that if I got near the four-hour mark and left the bubble, I would not be able to get back in fully and so would have to end the session.

The first song that had a significant effect on me was Henryk Gorecki, Symphony No.3, Op. 36. The second was Johannes Brahms: Ein Deutsches Requiem, Op.45.

I was sure that I had recorded my experiences when these songs were playing, but sadly somehow, the recorder was not turned on.

In the Symphony No. 3 piece, I recall going into a heavenly bliss state that I had been in before. I paid close attention to how it felt, and came up with words such as extreme bliss, carefree, vibratory, happy. It also had the standard "complete acceptance you feel in the moment as your ego disappears into pure gratitude for being alive." (I tend to say thank-you a lot during sessions.) People with a better grasp of the English language would have come up with better adjectives. This is the best I could do.

What happened in the Ein Deutsches piece, is that I ended up at one of the late crescendos in a blissful state, which also seemed to have some structure. It was a peak feeling experience. It occurred to me that this was the most important thing I had ever possessed, even though I knew how strange this would sound to an outsider.

While thinking about it, I realized that I could/would have when I am no longer part of this physical world. All my physical possessions, family, and friends would be gone, but this "feeling" I would still own.

This feeling was so amazing that I replayed the song again after it was over. It was stronger the second time, so I quickly recorded the experience on my audio recorder. But, there was nothing on the recording for some unexpected and unknown reason when I went to review it later.

Going back into the bubble, I played it a third time, and although the same valuable feeling arose at the same point in the song, it was not quite as strong as the second time around. It came to be one of the most exciting things I have ever experienced in my dozen high-dose sessions.

Lastly, the whole Session #13 left me incredibly happy. The same word occurred over and over during my entire session. The term was *profound.* I was not even sure what the word meant or how it applied. This led me to believe the word was being given to me as I don't recall ever using it in a sentence. I just kept repeating that this was the most profound experience of my life.

A couple of days after the trip, I went to the internet and looked to see if others had used the word profound related to their psilocybin experience. I found that it was commonly used. One example was in a statement by Katherine MacLean, one of the researchers working on the psilocybin work being performed at Johns Hopkins University. She stated, "Many years later, people are saying it was one of the most profound experiences of their life."

Session 14

This was the message I felt moved to post on Facebook as I was coming out of this session:

So, here's a story. Take it for what it is worth. I am 1 hour 48 minutes in, and although I have had three previous dances with this particular partner, this time there is nothing, and I mean nothing...

I lay down for the long wait until the session comes to an end. While lying there in a whiny mood, I said, "Take the booster. Ya never know."

I do it, and within seconds, all hell breaks loose. It was seconded. I am the luckiest person ever to walk the planet. Once I realize what is going on, I grab my tape recorder, which was ready (to record the lesson for the day) for moments like this, and I can't find it.

I then sense, 'you don't need the tape recorder. You won't remember much of this, but sit back and watch.' Went on for hours.

The luckiest man ever. You say you saw a better hand, I call, and all my chips are in.

That's a joke as to how would one know? That's just the way it made me feel—luckiest guy ever to walk the face of the Earth.

I was dealing with some sort of force in charge. As you can see from the above message written about six hours into the trip, I was very confident that I had been exposed to things others had not seen.

I also realized that by not recording, I would forget all but the overall feeling of being given knowledge and being incredibly grateful for seeing it. Also, I was left with the basic understanding that *the force* behind our reality creation was reasonable, but there are rules and that pain, suffering, and death are part of our evolution.

Things are born and die, and that is natural. We can also manifest great negativity such as war or death from alcohol or cigarettes through free will. Based on my encounter, I was convinced that all would work out in the end.

It seemed that I was experiencing a transcendent experience equivalent to the one Bill W. had that led him to start AA (Alcoholics Anonymous), or a mystical enlightenment experience like the Apostle Paul had on the road to Damascus. The sense of gratitude that I felt was beyond words.

Surveys from people at Johns Hopkins University seem to back up the fact that this almost divine *wow* slap in the head is experienced by many who have taken high-dose psilocybin. Seventy percent of all the people in the Johns Hopkins study stated that it was one of the top five experiences of their life, equivalent to the birth of a child or the death of a parent, and this feeling lasted long after their session.

The feeling of being in a Samadhi or Nirvana-type feeling was so strong that I kept joking that it appeared they were getting me ready to go out and start a new religion. After what I experienced, I can easily understand how people could start a religion after such an event.

Act 1 – Charlie's Angels

T here were absolutely no colors or shapes going into this experience. As usual, I didn't want lights, shapes, or dancing bears, just the lesson. As before, it went from absolutely nothing to a full-on trip.

From what I recall, the session started with the idea of Charlie's Angels. People who have followed my social media pages will know that I have three young female assistants who help me produce the YouTube channel, publish and co-author books, or conduct interviews.

Although no one says anything, I am sure everyone wonders how and why this situation exists. For some reason, in this high-dose session, that is where the lesson began.

The three young women, Desta Barnabe, Sinead Whelehan, and Nicole Sakach, are all about the same age and have come to be known as Charlie's Angels – three good-looking women taking instruction from some old guy.

In this experience, like many high-dose sessions, I go into a powerful flow state where I can see issues very clearly, and where answers (that appear to come as knowledge as opposed to just good ideas) come quickly. The only drawback is that all the emotion and most of the information fade when the session is over like a dream upon awakening.

What I was shown is that this situation may have been more synchronistic than I imagined. I thought having these women help me was based on my efforts to help younger people in the field, as I had done with young male researchers who I called the 'young guns,' because they worked so hard and appeared to be able to operate with computers and social message sites that had left most older researchers lost and out of touch.

What was impressed upon me was that I had not chosen them at all. All three of the ladies had approached me, and all of them I had met or interviewed, and then basically ignored them until they made a second attempt to get me to answer their emails. Once the second connection was made, each relationship took off.

I was shown a situation where beauty, power, and younger researchers who wanted to contribute, plus my dislike of technology and doing interviews, all played off each other to create success.

It appeared that having these ladies involved in the interviews enabled me to get interviews I would never be able to get. On the other hand, they would not have been in talks with some of the top people in the field without me.

Most importantly, two of them wanted to conduct interviews. All were able to operate efficiently in the social media world. All three were University educated. All were UFO experiencers who understood the consciousness connection. All had goals that they wanted to achieve in the field.

I was shown clearly that piles of things were brought to the table and that each needed the other to advance the message. Mostly, it showed me that it was in no way an accident. I would be nowhere without them, and they would be much less able to achieve their aspirations without me.

It was kind of a weird way to start a high-dose session, but that is what happened.

Act 2 – Oneness and Vibration

My experience has led me to believe that anyone using Penis Envy mushrooms should know how to deal with the left brain and fear. This strain can show bliss, but also hell. The only three "bad" moments I have ever had during my trips were on these mushrooms. Therefore, I went into this session very guarded to be aware of slipping down the rat hole.

Probably these mushrooms enormously aid in whatever is being mind-manifested. If the person taking them tries to control the experience or allows fear to enter, things can get ugly. (Sessions #11, #12, and #13 tell the story of what can happen.)

This session was comprised of a powerful Oneness experience. It did take me a few seconds to figure out what was happening. First, I sensed a feeling of bliss. It was as if I was moving up a mountain. The higher I got, the more blissful it became. Still, I had the impression that I was balancing on a bike and that any small slip would cause a state of darkness, loss of control, feeling the pain of dying people, or the seeing death and destruction all around me. It felt like these things were merely one thought away.

As I rose, I needed to maintain my balance so that when the Oneness experience began to happen, I thought that I was slipping into some negative manifestation. I do not recall most of what happened, but I felt that I was being pulled and twisted around. Naturally, I was resisting.

Then, I started to see that things were being pulled. It was similar to watching everything around me being stretched like a giant plastic toy. My impression was that this would turn into some weird B-movie, where people would start emerging with their faces melting off.

As this was happening and I was trying to balance rather than fight it, which is never good, I found myself looking at a plastic world where thoughts could change things, unlike our 3D, conscious world where we think everything is stable and unchangeable.

Realizing that something was being shown to me, I relaxed and saw a most impressive display of Oneness.

In recent weeks, I had watched many lectures by cognitive neuroscientist Donald Hoffman. He states that we cannot see reality. What we see is an icon in between us and ultimate reality. An example would be the steering wheel used in a video game. It is not the objective reality we think it is. Hoffman explains:

> *If you play the video game Grand Theft Auto with a virtual-reality add-on, you see a 3D world with 3D objects, such as a black steering wheel in front of you. If you turn your head, however, the steering wheel disappears. Indeed, it ceases to exist because it only exists when looking where it should be in the*

simulation. The reality that exists—circuits and software again—is utterly unlike a steering wheel. But it prompts you to create a steering wheel when needed and to destroy it when it isn't.

Therefore, what I was shown was an icon or symbol of the ultimate reality of Oneness. This is the first time a lesson on this topic was given to me. Many people have been shown Oneness, but each is shown a different analogy of the lesson. My assistant Sinéad Whelehan, for example, had a view of the Oneness experience during an Ayahuasca session in Peru. This is how she described it:

> *I could not see anything, but coming out from underneath my body were all these glowing lines. White glowing lines that were coming out from where I was sitting in space that was going out forever and ever, like, endlessly in every direction around me. These lines were crossing other lines, and where every line met, there was a dot of really bright, glowing, multicolored light.*
>
> *So, it is like I am sitting on a grid in the universe, and I'm thinking, 'Wow, this is amazing.'*

The space around us that we think is empty was portrayed as a substance like water but was not water. It looked like some mesh that had the consistency of water and could move like water. Everything was inside this meshy fluid, and when I moved or spoke, the mesh would move or vibrate, and the vibration would extend out everywhere. In the same way, any movement by anything around me would influence me. This seemed to even extend to things like sunlight. Everything was in a very plastic state and anything that happened vibrated into everything else. What I was sensing was fantastic, and it was at this point that I felt around for the audio recorder thinking, "I have to document this vision."

Again, I could not find the audio recorder and got the impression that I would not remember it all. Moreover, the second part of the lesson was now occurring. This part had to do with the vibration in the Oneness scenario. It was clear that everything was vibrating and that nothing was effectively static and unchanging. Somehow everything in the universe was constantly changing and affected by the vibration of everything around it.

This model fits an earlier noetic idea that I received in 2017, which said, *No nouns.* Nouns are created by the left brain that believes in objects and separation of those objects. What I was told then was that there are no objects. Matter is just one giant verb that is growing, and learning, and changing. Similarly, the human body contains 90 million cells that die every minute, and 90 million different cells are replacing the dead cells. The human body is continually changing every second.

This idea also fits with earlier encounters I had *the force.* In looking for words to describe it, all were verb-type objects, moving, creating, and swirling. There was no clear shape or form. The closest description would be a massive, powerful hurricane that was creating rather than destroying.

What was shown to me was a clear correlation with how Oneness and vibration work. Unfortunately, much of it disappeared like a dream. However, I was left with the certainty that I had been given what William James described as "insight into depths of truth unplumbed by the discursive intellect."

Act 4 - Luckiest Man Alive

Again, I was left many times during the experience feeling incredibly grateful for life and for what I learned during my 14th session. The only drawback was that I knew that much of this gratitude would be lost when Returning to the conscious world.

Forgetting is the usual pattern. William James (in describing mystical experiences) stated they last "at most an hour or two. That seems to be the limit beyond which they fade into the light of common day." I was even told during my trip that I would not remember. I was content not to record it and just watch since talking into an audio recorder pulls me out of the deep state where all the action is.

The snow globe was repeatedly shaken during the session. It was much more intense than any previous session as if the lessons were getting more complex and closer to a college level.

The height of gratitude came at around the four-hour mark, where I always seem to come out of a full bubble state and then must work at keeping it going. After four hours, I must concentrate intensely on the music, which will pull me back in. Before the four-hour mark, there is a sense of being locked into the experience, and it is difficult to think of anything else.

As the session came to a close, I heard the playlist's last three songs: *Gracious A La Vida*, *Swing Low Sweet Chariot*, and *What a Wonderful World*. The mood was set for giving thanks and the realization that it is a wonderful world.

At the end of the four hours, my flow state continued. Even though I could not wholly become one with the music, I could still think about things and get clear answers to my questions. This went on for another four hours where it was impossible to shut down my mind and go to sleep.

Although I could not remember too much, it was as telling as any revelation given to anyone. As with previous sessions, the information seems so essential that I considered going out to start a religion. Indeed, I thought whoever was behind the information was not going to make me do this.

I was left with a great sense of reverence for what I had been shown and forgotten, but the underlying emotion and belief in a world that is entirely under control remained. EVERYTHING is perfect in the world. Whoever is running the show has it all under control, and everything is perfect. Despite how fearful much of society is about the future, I felt confident that this fear was nothing more than the workings of the left-brain, conscious mind that spends all day worrying about life.

Session 15 – The Hallucination

Act 1

G oing into this session, I decided not to use the audio recorder, which was keeping me from going deeper into the field. This could be thought of as stopping an analytical overlay, as in Remote Viewing, where the left brain tries to take over the session and guess at the target. The left brain creates noise that does not allow the individual's right brain to pick up the signal in the field.

I took 3 grams of a new strain of mushrooms called McKennaii Magic Mushrooms to see if I would have a different experience. My trusty blindfold went on; I got my playlist ready and waited for the sensations to begin.

Like in Session #14, nothing happened, and I was already in over 2 hours. There were no vibrations, no colorful images, and no becoming One with the music. Frustrated and not wanting to kill the night, I took a 0.75-gram booster that I had placed on the desk, just in case. I swallowed it, put the blindfold back on, and got under the covers again.

In Session #14, the experience began only seconds after taking the booster. This time it took only a few minutes to kick in.

It started as other encounters had, with a vibration taking over my body. The vibration came mostly from my legs, and it was powerful in the upper part of my legs and groin. I worried that I would have to deal with the bathroom situation again where instead of going into the experience, I would be stuck in the physical world of trying to use the bathroom.

As with all sessions where an audio recorder was not used, I remember only a small part of what occurred. The first thing was the fight over the ego. After that, I don't know much of what happened.

The experience did become very intense. I sometimes refer to this as turbulence. It enters into at least 50% of the sessions. I experience the outlines of shapes lit up in beautiful and unique, fluorescent, psychedelic colors. I also get the surrender experience where objects come very close to me, almost as if it is testing my surrender reaction.

Act 2

At one point, I was in the flow state, and there was a back and forth with whatever is on the other side. I asked, "Am I hallucinating?"

The response was, "Of course, it's a hallucination, and you are living in it, you idiot." Part of what they showed me came as a sort of 'flight demo' about how reality is set up. I remember it was a challenging and scary ride, like a plane experiencing severe turbulence during a landing. There was a lot of uncertainty, and I thought that I might not make it this time. It was evident that during a trip, people have no idea what they are up against.

The force behind the experience always appears neutral to me. Rules are all set up and how you react to the rules determines how well you do. It comes across like a video game; the more you practice, the better you become. It isn't the video game that is evil, despite the number of people who swear at it while playing.

There are no shortcuts. There is no "I'm too sick to go to school today" – it is more like "Santa knows when you are sleeping" yada, yada. People who think they are brilliant geniuses will be crushed like a bug.

I believe that I am the luckiest person to walk the Earth. *The force* leaves you always assuming you are someone special being shown things that others have not seen.

Session 16

A gain, I did not record the entire experience. Therefore, much of what happened is gone to the world where lost dreams go. However, I did stop the session on several occasions because what seemed to be happening was so significant, and I knew if I didn't record it, the event and the emotion would be lost.

The psychedelic state has often been described as a rapid but uncontrolled trip into the field. What I concluded from this one was:

- The more sessions I do, the more information can be gathered. It is almost as if, after so many sessions, I have learned the dance steps. There are still reservations going in, knowing that surrender must take place and trying to take control can easily cause a gruesome trip. Everything except what I see and experience is pretty much predictable.
- Honestly, it seems that the more sessions I do, the deeper I can get in, the more I seem to be shown, the more the emotional reactions are to the events.

This time I used almost 4 grams to ensure there wasn't a repeat of my previous trip.

No colors and shapes were moving around going into the trip. These colors always occur at the beginning as if you are on a psilocybin plane moving through the clouds of colors and shapes to get to cruising altitude.

What I did experience going in was tremendous vibration. It started in the groin area and was causing the back of my thighs to spasm. This may be an essential factor because abductees will describe vibration in their body as they think they are being taken. It may eventually confirm that there is only one thing, and it is here and now. As John Wheeler declared, "there is no out there out there." We are not going anywhere. We may simply be changing our vibration, which puts us into another vibration (dimension/level/world). This again portrays the classic abductee story where they explain being taken through their bedroom wall or ceiling as they are taken to the craft.

Two stories in the real world seem to point to this idea that we are only going into ourselves, that what is happening is just an action inside consciousness, and that we only exist in the here and now, and everything is connected.

1. The famous artist, Akiane Kramarik, talked about an experience she had when she was five and disappeared. Her family, friends, and police searched for her for over 6 hours. In recounting the story, Akiane talks about being taken on a tour of the universe by an orb that gave off a Godlike sense. She reported "splitting into a myriad of fragments, hundreds upon hundreds of eyes that could see in all directions and participate in many

imperative planetary and extra-planetary proceedings all at the same time." Yet, at the same time, she stated she did not physically go anywhere. "I was able to see," she wrote, "exactly how many police officers, state troopers, firemen, search dogs, and neighbors were looking for me because of a suspected kidnapping; however, nobody could see me. That's right. Nobody."

2. The second story is an entirely unknown posting done by Ron Pandolfi, who has been rumored to be the man in charge at the CIA for all things paranormal. He has often hinted that the UFO story's truth lies in portals and gateways to other realities that are right here in our time and space. Here is what he wrote in 2015:

Why look for visitors when we are in their home? Why look for assistance from those who created the problem? The existing roadway does not define the pathway. Open a new door. Climb up a new staircase. Step into a new dimension. The Vectors are pointing from the past along established pathways. They cannot be stopped, but they can be bent. Drop a black hole and let the new world begin.

Act 1

People think that it is the type of music and the artist that are important. I am sure that what's most important is the vibration and the emotion of the music that is effecting the triggering. Even the stillness in between songs can be unnerving. Silence seems to have a vibration that causes me to become a bit fearful the longer it continues.

When a reflective piece is played, the participant's mind reflects to events in their life. These will be memories of people, happy/sad events, and places. A thought related to the past event pops into your consciousness, similar to having a therapist talking to someone about a troubling event in their past. The advantage in the psilocybin state is that the emotions are jacked up to full volume, and the "dealing with the issue" is done in the open with the high emotion "getting it all out." When the song ends, one is left with the feeling that the event has now been neutralized.

One reflective event that happened was that I had lost four people to the Covid situation, and they started to emerge as a group. I was able to reflect on the time I had with all of them. They appeared as a group, and the people I knew best were in the front and the others in the back. I knew Angelia Joiner the best, and she was in the front.

I also knew that I could go back with them and experience the pain of those around them, as opposed to their pain. It was a very emotional, tear-filled moment, almost like I had my own memorial service. The part that is impossible to convey is how real and highly emotional the moment becomes. It is beyond words and must be experienced.

This memorial moved to each of the people who had died of Covid. Again, I was flooded with the sadness and pain of those left behind. The scene changed to other people around the world dying for any other reason. Again, it was the pain of the people who had loved and known the deceased.

When the song was over, it was as if a fever had broken. The memories and the experience of mourning left me feeling grateful.

Act 2

I have audio of something I described as the most reverent, spiritual event of my life. It was one of the circumstances whereby focusing intently on the music allowed my consciousness to soar upwards. The higher the awareness ascended, the more intensely blissful the experience was. Bliss was somehow related to the vibration, and focused attention will increase the emotion, vibration, and joy many times.

Unusually this time, I experienced the overwhelming feeling of relevance. Strangely, I felt that the sensation was some fluid or substance, and I was being drenched in it. I cannot think of any life experience that can describe accurately how intense this was. I kept thinking, "I didn't know reverence was a thing."

Act 3

Another song and more mind wandering.

It is crucial to record mind wanderings under the influence. The idea came to me and pointed out that this might not be the same "little voice in the head" as what we perceive while in the conscious world.

We know from the physical world that the little voice is our left-brain, ego talking. It tends to be into self, pointing out all the fearful things that can attack it, leaving you feeling insecure and unworthy. It over-analyzes, makes you rehash old problems repeatedly, makes you feel like you aren't good enough, and prevents you from ever getting started.

The difference in the psilocybin experience is that the default mode network (DMN) has shut down under the influence. More importantly, the brain rewires itself, and now parts of the brain that do not usually talk are directly communicating. There is a lot of cross-talk between the left and right brain.

This means that we cannot employ physical, typical brain models in the session because the regular brain network is shut down. You have a completely different brain until the session is over.

I am in what I call a flow state. I experienced the same state in 2012 and 2017 when I had clear, noetic experiences. A feeling identifies it. It has a sense of certainty that the information coming is knowledge, and it is time to find a paper and pen and then write as quickly as possible.

While in this flow state, I can ask a question or think about something, and answers come like lightning bolts. Everything seems more transparent, and the information coming has that sense of certainty. I started to pay close attention to the fleeting thoughts realizing this communication might be coming from "Mr. Smart" instead of the conscious voice from the left brain, often identified as "Mr. Stupid."

Act 4

I have been shown images that describe how reality works. It is not actually reality, but the interface to reality, which says, "reality of something like this." I now agree with those researchers who believe there is no way to see reality accurately. The critical analogy that is used to illustrate this is that you have an icon on your desktop for email, but it is not the email. It is just an interface that we use.

One of the lessons I came to understand was the idea of memory. The way it was shown to me was as a giant horizontal spiderweb extending out from every person. Every memory was stored in this spider web and linked by subject. When a person starts thinking about something, the awareness would need to access the memories in the spider's web to compose the thought.

I saw that as a person has a thought, the memory of that piece of information would light up in a part of the spider web. A large red glow would travel up to the person that seemed like it was at the speed of light. This idea was that the memory was sent to the person, not the other way around. It was almost like the memory was as alive as the person.

Therefore, if I were to ask, "Who was your first boyfriend/girlfriend?" Immediately in your awareness, the answer would appear. Where did that memory come from? It seemed to me that the memory says, "Here I am," and races into your conscious awareness. It is all occurring inside consciousness, and it's all linked.

Act 5

An overwhelming emotion that struck me was reverence. I never think about it in daily life, but it was the dominant feeling in this session.

Another fantastic emotion was gratitude. It, like the reverence, felt like it was something that was taking over my thoughts. I felt this gratitude for what I was experiencing in the session and also in life. It made me think that I was the luckiest person in the world. It was as if I had been shown things and felt things that others did not have access to. It seemed that if I left life at this moment, I could tip my hat and say, "I'm ready to go. That was a good life."

Act 6

One of the most significant events of the whole night was the forgiveness event. One of these occurred in an earlier session, where I placed all of my failings and sins on a table in front of some powerful force.

This time the feeling was more like I was being forgiven for everything. It was a strong feeling that occurred a few times during the night. There were two that I faintly recall:

1. Whatever it was, it came in from the side and did the forgiveness like a mother hovering in front of me and fixing a cut. I could hear the words. "There, all better now. Do you feel better?" It sounded like it was talking to me as a young child.

2. The second was very bizarre. There was a song that had both male and female choral sections. The male singers tend to produce a strong but darker feeling. The female singers (especially soprano opera singers) can create soaring, blissful moments. When one is about to build up to a crescendo, I have to focus hard on the music, and it is like taking a high-speed elevator up. This song had both parts, and I did not want to focus on the darker section lest I start to manifest some negative image (sometimes it is like being on a bicycle balancing between the dark and light vibrations). I was attempting to grab the dark music and pull it up with the soaring female music.

As I did, everything shifted for me; looking up at sort of a box structure, I heard the words, "You're healed." I immediately thought, "Healed from what? I didn't want to be healed. I didn't ask for this."

Then the intense feeling of being in a forgiveness oven took place. Like gratitude, forgiveness felt like it had substance. As this was going on, I was thinking, "Well, we'll see if the two small physical problems get healed." (They were not.) It was a very bizarre experience.

Act 7

After four hours, the intense dancing bears part is over. I am back in the hallucinatory reality, yet my mind is still in a flow state, as long as I keep the headset on with the music playing.

In this flow state, the memories and thoughts move through the spider web much quicker. It almost feels like there is no resistance to thought. I think about something, and things are flashing by me, almost like answers to a question. This flow state can go on for hours.

This time I asked some questions to see if it would give me some noetic wisdom. I was about to provide an online lecture, and the hot topic in the UFO community is always disclosure. I asked, and nothing happened. I focused and asked again.

Then I sensed the answer, "Who cares?" I also got the sense that it was saying, "Why do you ask," and then either "You asked this already" or "You know the answer to this." It was like I knew better and should not have even asked.

To sum up the answer, it doesn't matter what the government or anyone in the government thinks about the UFO issue. This is a question of why I came into this world. I should be busy with my newly found mission of investigating consciousness and stop bringing up what others are doing or thinking. We all agreed to come into this world to do something. When we die, we get asked one question, "How did you do? You set up the play. How did it work out?". What people think or do doesn't matter.

It was giving me the line that every parent has given to their child. Everyone has probably had the experience of a child wanting to do something like stay out until midnight at 16 years old. When the child is told No, the child replies, "My friends are allowed to." To which you reply, "I don't care what your friends do. They don't make the rules around here."

Children are susceptible to what their friends do and think. They do not want to be rejected. They want to fit it.

Disclosure is like that. We want to find someone who will permit us to believe. We are interested in what others think as if that belief will bolster our fragile ego.

What will we do if the government does come out and say it is all real? We will do nothing, just as no one did anything after the New York Times and the Washington Post announced that the government was studying UFOs after denying it for 51 years. People didn't do anything because it had nothing to do with them. They still had to go to work, feed their family, and take the kids to soccer practice.

Act 8

In the flow state after the four hours, asked about UFOs to see what I would get back. What I got was an addition to something I had already talked about. That is my theory of WOW. The theory postulates that everything the intelligence behind the UFO phenomena does is simply done to make us go WOW and question the reality around us.

Why are the aliens are here, and what are they doing here? It's not an accident. There is an intelligence that is trying to break us out of this 3D reality. It is using other phenomena such as paranormal activities to wake us up to it.

The intelligence is also using the 'trickster phenomenon' where an entity flaunts the typical societal expectations to jar the people to throw them out of their everyday perceptions of reality.

As I thought about it, two of the elements of my theory of WOW popped up:

1. UFO sightings are witnessed to help us realize we are not alone and that something strange is going on that needs an explanation. UFOs make zig-zag patterns in the sky, not because they need to zig-zag around for any reason, but to make the people watching go WOW, because it is something that we on Earth cannot do. It makes us think there is something bigger than us out there.

2. In the same way, they drop small pieces of metal (metamaterials) or crash their saucers to alert us that something paranormal is taking place. They will drop metal and metal in which the isotopes have been altered because they know this will make the researchers have a meltdown.

The point became clear. The paranormal doesn't make sense. Yet, it must be following the laws of the universe. Instead of telling each other weird paranormal stories, we should stop and say, "Take a closer look. What is it really?"

Act 9 – The Reflection

In many of my experiences, I have come up against *the force*. It has no form. The best to describe what I see is that it is like a live, moving, and swirling cloud without edges.

In Session #16, I ran up against it again. Instead of coming off like male or female energy or an all-powerful force, this time, it came across like a long-time friend. My initial reaction was, "Oh, there you are." I felt instantly comfortable and at ease.

Usually, I recognize it immediately, but this time it started a bit different. I was moving from right to left, and it was on the other side as if there was some gap or river between.

While I was looking at this sort of cloud-type thing, it appeared either upset or angry, as if it was a storm cloud forming. I backed away, and the anger element left. It was *the force* that was reflecting my feeling, and when I stopped, it instantly disappeared.

Moving to the left, I presented another feeling, and it mimicked my feeling. Suddenly, I had moved to the right, and there on the other side of whatever was a mirror. I could see my face in it and immediately knew what the lesson had been.

It is the story told by the channeler Bashar who said:

If you look in a mirror and see your reflection is frowning, you don't go over to the mirror and try to make the reflection smile- you know that the only way to get the reflection to smile is to decide to smile first.

Same, physical reality is not outer; it is inner; it's just a reflection of you at every given moment, individually and collectively. So, if you wish to change your outer physical reality, all you really need to do is change something about yourself, and you will see that change take place unerringly and effortlessly.

Holotropic Breath Work

Holotropic breathwork is a technique developed by Stanislav Grof and his wife. This method is essential to study with its correlation to psychedelics because it can attain similar non-dual states without any drug being used. The only technique that is applied is the breath.

In his book, *The Holotropic Mind: The Three Levels of Human Consciousness and How They Shape Our Lives,* Grof wrote:

> *The key experiential approach I now use to induce non-ordinary states of consciousness and gain access to the unconscious and superconscious psyche is Holotropic Breathwork, which I have developed jointly with Christina over the last fifteen years. This seemingly simple process, combining breathing, evocative music, and other forms of sound, bodywork, and artistic expression, has an extraordinary potential for opening the way for exploring the entire spectrum of the inner world.*

Holotropic breathing invalidates the whole chemical theory that non-dual states of consciousness are just the brain on drugs. There is no drug in holotropic breathing, indicating that a simple breathing technique can shut down the left, survival part of the brain to stop it from creating our 3D world just as effectively as a psychedelic. Both breathing and psychedelics can shut down the part of the brain that creates the hallucinatory 3D world. Both allow the right brain to access higher states of consciousness. Grof often spoke of remembering that the conscious mind constructs the 3D world:

> *Consciousness does not just passively reflect the objective material world; it plays an active role in creating reality itself.*

Shortly after doing Session #4, I tried again to do holotropic breathwork, which uses deep breathing and other elements to allow access to non-ordinary states of consciousness. Dr. Stanislav Grof studied LSD and other psychedelics in Prague in the early 1950s. In 1973 he and his wife developed Holotropic breathwork, a type of psychotherapy, in California.

Like the sensory deprivation tank and meditation, I had tried holotropic breathwork in the past without success on my own. Those who promote these procedures have certainly been successful, especially if they are extroverts or have the extra money to attend a course on the subject. Like many others, I prefer to work alone, regardless of the fears I may encounter since it is clear to me that fear that our ego identifies is simply a pattern we have grown to accept.

I sat up one night trying to do the breathing. It is a process of basically forcing oneself to hyperventilate. I watched a YouTube video with a shortened form of the technique, calling for 10 minutes of heavy breathing and then following the body's instructions as to what to do next. It was hard to do for ten minutes, so I ended up falling asleep. The feeling when I woke was strange. Looking at the clock, it appeared that I had been asleep much longer than I thought possible.

Trying again, I continued the breathing and found that it was much easier to do lying down. I was able to go much longer and wasn't thinking, "When will this end?" After a few minutes, there was a cool sensation around my head, like a fan was pointed at me.

Focusing on the coolness, I wondered how this could be happening when I realized that my awareness was now focused on the experience. This was an epiphany. My impression was this was what people must be talking about when discussing that they are "awake and aware during meditation." This, to me and others, has always been easier said than done, and I would usually find my monkey mind off thinking about something else.

This was different. My consciousness was glued to the experience of what was happening to my body. It was like a precise and controlled meditation.

I picked up the breath and started to feel the tingling sensation in my arms and legs, then instructed my body to breathe some more quick breaths while my awareness stepped back to observe.

Unfortunately, this attempt was made so late that I could no longer stay awake, so stopped and was asleep almost immediately.

The next morning, I decided to try this breathing during my next psilocybin session while waiting for the medicine to work its magic. It would be a similar practice to Terence McKenna, who would meditate, waiting for the experience to begin.

Microdosing

The basic concept of microdosing is nothing new. Albert Hofmann, who first synthesized LSD in 1938, considered it one of the drug's most promising and least researched applications. He was among the first to realize its antidepressant and cognition-enhancing potential, [vi] famously taking between 10 and 20 µg himself, twice a week, for the last few decades of his life.
-Paul Austin

As a part of my search for answers, I studied and partook in a microdose phase of my investigation. This was done after talking to people in a psychedelics group where many were doing it.

In the past, I had tried but did not notice any change. As everyone in the group talked about positive results, I decided to do it through capsules sold by a company where everything was controlled and measured.

My first session began at the end of September using what is called the Fadiman protocol:

1. Day 1 – Dose 500mg capsule taken at 3:00 pm. I also took 250 mg of niacin, which I take daily
2. Day 2 – Afterglow day where a person is supposed to feel good
3. Day 3 – Rest day where the body returned to normal
4. Day 4 - Dose 500mg capsule again

At 4:00 pm each day, I volunteer at a senior citizen facility. Because of Covid-19, I wear a mask. That is where I felt the first effects. I could sense my breath in and out inside the mask and thought this is weird. I must have imagined it as you should not feel anything when microdosing.

By the time I got home 45 minutes later, I was feeling the microdose. I sat and meditated, but it did not feel like my regular meditations. I started to wonder if I might have to cut the capsule next time, which could be messy.

After eating dinner, I noticed that it had been 2.5 hours since I took the microdose and that I would have to lie down. I put on the eyeshades and turned on the music. It was an enjoyable trip, but there were no images or messages. What I had taken was unquestionably not a standard microdose. That night I also had trouble sleeping, which often happened the night after sessions.

The next day, while listening to James Fadiman about micro-dosing, he brought up points that solved it. He mentioned that people reporting back on micro-dosing who took niacin reported that it increased the intensity of psilocybin. He also recommended microdosing before 10 am as psilocybin had a stimulant effect, and some people reported trouble sleeping.

In my next microdose sessions, I eliminated many of the side effects by dosing early in the day and avoiding niacin on dose days. There still was an effect from that, but I noticed that by dosing early and then by moving around and doing everyday things like going for coffee, I barely noticed. One strange effect that did remain was that I was aware of breathing in my mask while working.

Positive effects of stress and attitude were what others have reported. However, that did not interest me, and I found myself longing to go back to high dosage to be taught lessons about how reality worked. I resolved to try the microdose for 30 days, and then go back to regular psilocybin sessions.

My assistant, Desta Barnabe, has had her own experiences with microdosing psilocybin. She has written the rest of this chapter.

A few years ago I did some research on microdosing with both psilocybin and LSD and was quite taken by the results that people were reporting. A very informative TED Talk from Ayelet Walden, called *Microdosing: A really good day* was a great introduction into what this medicine could do for people with depression. This was intriguing as I knew many people with anxiety and depression who were desperate and I wanted more information that might help them. I watched Paul Stamets' microdosing lectures and he has brought to light many studies on different types of mushrooms and their health benefits on illnesses like cancer.

Psilocybin is not addictive and in essence change the biochemistry of your mind. This allows it to be helpful in depression, anxiety, and obsessive-compulsive disorders. Mushrooms are virtually non-toxic and appear to be a very powerful psychotherapeutic drug.

When the brain it is being microdosed it is breaking addictive patterns. A cyclic pattern is created in the brain, for example, when an alcoholic reaches for another drink after they encounter an upsetting feeling. This cycle is a repetitive detrimental pattern that needs to be broken. Someone with Obsessive Compulsive Disorder or OCD, might feel anxious about getting sick from germs and will wash their hands or do a counting ritual to protect themselves. Again, this is a destructive, repeating pattern in the brain that could be eliminated by introducing tiny doses of psilocybin.

A good friend of mine was drinking a lot daily. He had been doing this for years and was caught up in a pattern of self-medicating by consuming alcohol. I told him about these microdosing studies, and he was interested in trying it out, though he was not hopeful that it would work. After following the 3-month protocol, he hasn't drunk for two years and counting.

Another friend had significant anxiety problems. He was constantly worried that he was sick and had some severe health problems. There would be a new problem every month, but for years he had not been able to break away from thinking that he had new symptoms of some unknown illness, usually cancer, that would kill him. This caused him to experience panic attacks, insomnia, and constant anxiety.

He, too, decided to try microdosing. After two months on it, he reported many similar revelations as I did when I took it myself. He experienced a closer connection to his dreams, a general decrease in over-thinking, a significant reduction in concern over his health, an increase in the duration of sleep, and a *lighter* feeling overall like he had had an enormous weight lifted off of him. His girlfriend reported that he was like a completely different person, he was returning to the person she knew over a decade ago when he was more carefree and fun to be around.

Another friend had a compulsive cleaning "habit." She also tried the protocol and felt she really "loosened up" her compulsion to have her environment so clean, orderly and organized. She also noticed less desire to eat desserts all night as she watched TV.

Many other friends I have shared this information with who hoped to see some benefits from microdosing, and who followed the protocol were pleased with the results.

For myself, I didn't have any addictions or patterns that I needed to break. I wanted to do the protocol to see if I would experience any right-brain effects, and I certainly did.

I noticed that my dreams and memories were being affected. When I would also smoke cannabis, vivid memories which I would never have been able to recall in waking reality would pop up. As the memory resurfaced, I would relive the experience as if I was there again in real-time. For some reason, memories of when I travel usually come up. I was in India and walking down a dusty street where I had once been. I could see what I was wearing and see my feet in my sandals; I would get in a rickshaw and remember exactly how much it costs and go to a beach which I had forgotten about because I didn't have any photos of it. I would feel the sweat on my face and sense the breeze and the smell of food cooking from a street vendor. Things would come up that I cannot recall myself anymore, but I would be right there and re-experience the entire memory.

Another thing I had a better recall with was dreams. I have a dream journal that I use to record strange dreams in. But again, after a couple of months of microdosing, as soon as I would smoke cannabis, I would instantly remember all my dreams from the night before, even if I had not remembered dreaming at all when I had awoken that morning. I felt as though the connection between my left brain and right brain was becoming more established, and they were finally sharing information better.

Another effect I encountered was eating less. This seemed unusual, and it took a month until I realized it could have been a result of the mushrooms. I had never heard of this, so when I found a Reddit thread where people were discussing this happening to them, I realized that it made sense. Eating was not an addiction for me, but I think what happened was that there might have been patterns when I was eating out of boredom or stress. Suddenly, I didn't think of eating as soon as I woke up or when I was bored at night. I ate when I was hungry and had no desire to eat if I wasn't.

Hopefully more money will be allocated into studying this plant medicine. Many people now can only find answers online and on Reddit discussion boards.

The protocol I have used and shared with others is:

The dosage is approximately 150 mg every three days. Even easier to remember is to take them twice a week on the same days every week, for example every Wednesday and Saturday. For the specific micro dosage, it is recommend is that you start taking 75 mg-100 mg. Each designated day after this, you up your dose 25 mg. when you come to the day where you can 'feel something.' This feeling is compared to having one too many coffees. Then you go back down 25 mg and use that amount going forward. You aren't supposed to feel anything when you are microdosing. You are just introducing the substance into your body. The average amount people settle on for their dosage is about 150-200 mg. I've heard from 250 lb male friends to 125 lb female friends, and they all roughly use about 150 mg. This protocol suggests dosing every three days for three months. then stopping completely. Assess your feelings for a few months. If you think you need another cycle, then do another 3-month protocol. Many people report that one 3-month cycle is all they need for years. If they start to feel any of those patterns reemerging, then begin the 3-month cycle again.

I do this cycle twice a year and this seems to keep these new connections with my right-brain healthy and active.

Observations

Is there any answer except that it comes from consciousness?
-John Wheeler

I n summing up what I took from my Psilocybin School is that it is a Contact Modality. Many other modalities can be used that will also produce the same non-ordinary mystical experiences. These would include ayahuasca, DMT, 5-MeO-DMT (5-methoxy-N, N-dimethyltryptamine), LSD, and many other non-chemical compound processes such as hypnosis, holotropic breathwork, and meditation.

Psilocybin, from my personal experience, is a shortcut to the enlightenment of actual reality. This fits right into our western "give me everything yesterday" mentality.

It can seem very uncontrolled because once the plant medicine is taken, there is no exit door. The subject will go wherever the psilocybin decides to go, and this can seem like a roller coaster ride where the coaster starts to disassemble mid-way through the trip.

Psilocybin seems to amplify both positive and negative emotions. If you were to take psilocybin and spend the day in nature, you might feel a stronger connection with her. If you were to be at a party and a fight broke out, you may be overwhelmed with fear, possibly leading to a bad trip.

Psilocybin, and other psychedelics, pull us out of the narrative we have built about reality. Materialistic science will say the experience is a hallucination, but that is just a word to keep the narrative alive that this is a real world.

During a breakthrough in a psilocybin experience, we discover that there is no time. This is what Albert Einstein described. He stated in 1955, just before his death, "To those of us who believe in physics, this separation between past, present, and future is only an illusion, if a stubborn one."

During the psychedelic experience, we learn that space is a function of the mind. Following the famous "spooky action at a distance" experiment with entangled particles, many folks like historian Richard Tarnas started to point out that space may not exist either. Tarnas stated that space and time could not be said to be characteristic of the world in itself, for they are contributed in the act of human observation. They are grounded epistemologically (in knowledge) like the mind, not ontologically (in existence) like things.[22]

The Great Race

Without consciousness, there is nothing... Consciousness is the central fact of your life.
-Neuroscientist Dr. Christof Koch

The psychedelic revolution of experimentation and research has in some ways become part of the capitalist health, wealth, and enlightenment movement. People set intentions to overcome fear, anxiety, PTSD, smoking cessation, or have a spiritual experience. In my case, the purpose is to collect more information. Psychedelics have become a powerful tool to accumulate more.

It is not that there is anything terrible about these intentions. However, it makes me laugh that it is about getting more. We in the west have more than people in poor third-world countries could even imagine. Many pushing the psychedelic issue have a well-paying job, big house, two cars, two kids, maybe a cabin at the lake.

We have got it all, but in a capitalist country that preaches more, we continually see the next bobble that leads to the ultimate happiness that seems just out of reach.

That may be the answer to why someone who has a billion dollars doesn't retire and enjoy the money. Once you have a billion, you need two billion in a world of collecting material stuff. The world has gotten so crazy that in recent discussions, it was mentioned that Jeff Bezos made 113 billion dollars in the eight months of the COVID-19 crisis. He now is worth 193.2 billion, even after a divorce, while many Americans lost their jobs, homes, and health care. The discussion was not, Is this enough for one man? Instead, it is on the speculation on who will be the first trillionaire.

In such a consumerist world, many are attracted to the paranormal and the spiritual, not so much for the answer to why we are here but as a form of entertainment.

People in the UFO community will pay $4,000 for a trip to the desert to hopefully see a UFO. People always ask me who would be so stupid to pay that amount of money. My reply is, "Lots of people." People want to see something physically. But when I bring up the mystical side of UFO experiences or the underlying message from the aliens, few seem to care.

That, I believe, is why all scientific, psychedelic research is tied to consumerism. It costs millions of dollars to run a double-blind study that allows doctors (if you can afford to go to one) the power to write a psychedelic prescription to cure you of whatever ails you.

An industry of producing pure psilocybin (since street mushrooms are portrayed as totally uncontrolled, unregulated, and potentially unsafe) has begun. Companies with big money funders have started to move in on a possibly deregulated future. It is costly, at $7,000 - $10,000 a gram in 2018 (13x mushroom street price), and all those who are handling it charge money to take it and do the paperwork.

Needed Resource	Cost	Final Billing
Therapists for Flight Instructions	$60-125/Hour 8 hours x 2 people	$960- 2,000
FIRST Dosing session	$60-125/ Hour 8 hours x 2	$960-2,000
SECOND Dosing Session	$60-125/ Hour 8 hours x 2	$960-2,000
Integration session After	$60-125/ Hour 8 hours x 2	$960-2,000
Pure Psilocybin	3x $135 x 2 sessions (2018 wholesale price)	$810
Director cost, room rental, Dr. on call, company profit	???	???

This would mean that the psilocybin cost for a 30mg/70kg dose would be around $405 wholesale in 2018 dollars. The retail price would run over $1,000 per session for the drug alone, and two sessions are usually recommended. The more you look at it, the more it seems like just a new Big Pharma play to deal with stockholders' bottom line. The first concern will not be the mind of the patient.

The regulations add high costs, such as at the NYU research lab where an 800 lb. safe was bolted to the floor.

Then FDA regulators forced the pharmacologists, who were researching it, to take out <u>one gram</u> every day, weigh it, and have witnesses to the daily process.

The future psychedelic world will clearly need many well-paid guides, psychiatrists, and therapists to do integration work.

Dr. Robin Carhart-Harris described the funding pitfall where it could end up behind a paywall, as compared with the present model where a physician spends 10 minutes and hands out a prescription for Prozac:

> *What are the subtle nuances that we need to think about...There are some potential complications to consider as well with the mass upscaling of psychedelics...my hope- the high-level thing to say- I hope there nothing prohibitive in terms of access pending the relevant level sensible safeguarding is in place? I really do not want cost to be prohibitive, and I hope there is a way to manage the rollout so that it's not. At the moment, the cost-effectiveness calculations to break that right down – how expensive this is for people, privately or through their insurance companies, or in public health-care systems, if this will be cheap enough to be integrated. That is one of the key problem areas.[23]*

People are selling psilocybin as a cure to this and that, and the proponents of the cures have websites, courses, and offers as guides or councilors for sale, which will guide people along the yellow brick road to the beautiful Land of Oz. Like the UFO example, when I talk about the free spiritual aspect, people's eyes sort of roll back in their head with disinterest.

Nice Story

Every complex problem has a solution that is simple, neat, and wrong.
-H. L. Mencken

The first principle is that you must not fool yourself, and you are the easiest person to fool.
-Dr. Richard Feynman

Reality is what we take to be true. What we take to be true is what we believe. What we believe is based upon our perceptions. What we perceive depends upon what we look for. What we look for depends on what we think. What we think depends on what we perceive. What we perceive determines what we believe. What we believe determines what we take to be true. What we take to be true is our reality.
-Prof David Bohm

Researchers have created many nice stories around what they believe accounts for the psilocybin and holotropic breath visions: (The keyword in the sentence being stories.)

Psilocybin rapidly metabolizes into psilocin, which like the neurotransmitter serotonin, binds with 5-H2A receptors in our brains. That blood flow and

249

oxygen content in our medial prefrontal and posterior cingulate cortices and our thalami areas, referred to as our default mode networks," appear to decrease when psilocin is facilitating the occurrence of alternate states of consciousness.[24]

Here is another story for hyperventilation that has a connection to holotropic breathing:

Relative to the bicarbonate concentration, the pH increases above normal because the bicarbonate concentration does not decrease as rapidly. The condition where the pH of the body is increased above normal is called "alkalosis," and all the body fluids and cells become more alkaline than normal. This effect lies on the basis of the mental effects of hyperventilation. So, what are the mental effects of hyperventilation?

This story is no different than the account of describing Moses as he parted the Red Sea. Moses gathers the children of Israel at the seashore and strikes the water with his staff. A great wind arises, and the sea opens up. The floor of the sea is dry, and the people walk through to the other side. When everyone is through, Moses taps his staff again, and the sea closes on the Egyptians who are chasing them.

The story is accurate, and it is a lovely story. It, however, leaves out explaining the miracle. How did Moses perform the trick that divided the sea? In the example of holotropic breathing, how do the conscious effects create the mystical vision? A description of pH rising does not explain consciousness. It is nothing more than a story of this happening, and when this occurs, then there is a miracle.

In the story told about psilocybin, there is an observation of decreased blood flow to the default mode network, which gives an individual a sense of ego. This creates the breakdown of the importance of individual self and the illusion of Oneness of all things. Like Moses at the Red Sea, scientists are merely describing the observed process that explains nothing.

The original story was that psychedelics caused increased blood flow in the brain, which caused more significant brain activity, which causes the illusions. Amanda Feilding at the British Beckley Foundation did research and discovered the story was wrong. To correct it, they just made up a new story.

The problem with the new default mode network story is that it is just a story and nothing more. It is solving a mystery with another enigma. It is merely saying A did this, then B did this, and C happened. It is a description of the event but explains nothing. A report is not an explanation, as in where an unenlightened neurologist hangs on to the story that psychedelic effects are just brain chemistry.

Who is causing the blood flow to increase in some areas and decrease in other areas? Blood flow is just blood flow. It is secondary to the mental event. The blood flow, EEG changes, and stimulation of serotonin 2A receptors (5-HT2ARs) by psilocybin's active metabolite psilocin are only correlated no differently from correlates found in a radio or a TV. The fMRIs show pretty pictures but explain extraordinarily little.

If we were to imagine someone finding a radio or TV 200 years ago, those investigating would see all sorts of things lighting up and responding as the sound or picture operates. It does not mean that the singer is on the radio or that there is a soccer game going on inside the TV.

A wonderful analogy of this storytelling of a complex system is the human cell division, which many still call "simple cell division." A new cell created in the human body now prepares to divide and create another new cell. A cell consists of 100 trillion atoms, which means that building the second cell must source the right 100 trillion new cells to build the new cell. We say simple cell division when we have no idea where it gets the atoms, how it picks them, and then moves them to the area where the new cell will be created. We replace the complex process with a story that "it gathers" when if we had to do it, we could not source the first ten atoms needed in the process.

A cell brings in the 100 trillion atoms at the right time and then puts them into the right three-dimensional spot in the correct order. We replace that complex process with the word divides. Nice story. Now explain how it is being done.

Does the cell have a brain that is the contractor for the building process? We counter that with DNA memory, which is just another story. We use one unexplained account to explain another unexplained story. The reductionist scientific method is doing nothing more than breaking one giant unexplained story into many smaller unexplained stories.

The new cell, which has never built a cell, can do the mitosis process in two hours. Like itself, the cell it creates has all the information necessary to construct another billion or trillion fully functioning humans. That is a description of the story. It may be good enough for scientists, but it explains nothing.

Those materialists who are making up the stories have been around for so many years have no clue how to build the new cell. They will claim they do and can show experiments in a lab with cell division. This, however, is taking credit for what the cell is doing. Build a cell without getting a cell to do it for you. At that point, we come to realize the story is no better than any story told to little children in Sunday School.[9]

Another example is the fact that the human body loses 300 million cells a minute. These cell deaths take place among 210 different cells. We can say that all 300 million cells are replaced for all 210 other cells in the right proportion at precisely the right time. To say the body does it explains nothing.

Materialist science has handled this brain consciousness dilemma by using the same process that was rumored to have been proposed by Richard Feynman, "shut up and calculate," to deal with the Copenhagen Interpretation of quantum mechanics. In short, this meant just to do the calculations in quantum mechanics to develop technology and avoid the underlying philosophical consciousness implications.

Another method used to bypass the mystery is to use placeholders. Give it a name, and that makes it go away. It is

---

[9] This is basically the message that I picked up from the Universe in Chapter 8, Act 3, where arrogant and ignorant people think they can explain reality, when in actuality they have not got a clue as to how it works.

just this process or that process. The most popular is that the inexplainable is only nature or evolution doing its thing. One might as well be giving credit to the three-fingered banana monkey.

The Copenhagen interpretation theory was proposed by Nobel Laureates Niels Bohr and Werner Heisenberg. It says that physical systems generally do not have definite properties before being measured by a conscious observer. Two other Nobel Laureates, John Von Neuman and Eugene Wigner added to that importance of consciousness in the process of the physical world, stating, "consciousness causes collapse."

Therefore, neurologists can describe all sorts of stories of what they think they see in the brain. Still, none of these stories avoids the underlying consciousness philosophical problem.

Feynman summed up the quantum physics observation stories saying, "If you think you understand quantum mechanics, you don't understand quantum mechanics."

In the same way, it could be said that if neurologists think they understand consciousness, they don't.

This does not stop materialists from promoting and teaching their dogma as a factual explanation. Max Planck's physics professor told him in 1874 to avoid studying theoretical physics since everything was already understood. Their bottom-line belief is I know, and you just believe.

In a paper produced by philosopher Neal Grossman in the Journal of Near-Death studies called "Who's Afraid of Life After Death," he recounts the story of a colleague who dismissed NDE as coincidences and lucky guesses. Grossman asked him what would convince him that NDEs were real. His colleague replied, "even if I were to have a near-death experience myself, I would conclude that I was hallucinating rather than believing my mind could exist independently of my brain."

Max Planck described the habit of scientists who believe stories and then defend them to the death, with his famous science advanced one funeral at a time, "A great scientific truth does not triumph by convincing its opponents and making them see the light, but rather because its opponents eventually die, and a new generation grows up that is familiar with it."

Contact Modality Crossovers

I described my first DMT experience with Terence McKenna back in 1986. It was an encounter with the beings. I was absolutely floored. You know they emerged out of a flaming waterfall; you know raging color. There are about half a dozen of them, three to four feet tall. They just kind of emerged out of this waterfall, and they chirped, or you know lilted, or you know whatever, telepathically spoke to me saying, "You know now. Do you see now? Do you see now? Do you see? That went on for a few minutes, and I came down and decided to study DMT.

-Dr. Rick Strassman, professor of psychiatry

One of the more interesting things I observed in looking at psilocybin and other psychedelic drugs is the parallel to other contact modalities where people use UFOs and meditation to get into the non-local field.

The most interesting is the entities seen in high-dose psychedelic excursions.

-People who do incredibly high doses of psilocybin (20+ grams) report running into the praying mantis beings with eyes as big as plates. Sid Goldberg told me he had an encounter with a praying mantis being while meditating.

-People who do very high-dose LSD, 5-MeO-DMT, or high-dose morning glory seed sessions, report seeing light beings. UFO abductees see the light beings (which is the #1 reported being). People like my assistant Sinead Whelehan also saw energy beings during an ayahuasca session.

-Machine elves are reported by those who ingest high dose psilocybin and DMT. Strassman was so concerned with how many people had seen aliens that he would ask the people in his 1990s DMT study if they had been abducted. Abductees report seeing small greys. Most importantly, I interviewed most of the people who had been in two xendras (portals) that opened up at Mount Shasta in 2014 and 2015. As part of that event, people described small alien beings hiding behind trees where they appeared to be smiling and playing a game of hiding and seek. When I asked the witnesses if they were greys, they said no. Most described them as looking like mischievous elves.

-One person who took DMT reported an experience that was almost identical to an alien abduction. "I felt like I was in an alien laboratory, in a hospital bed like this... A sort of landing bay or recovery area. There were beings. They had a space ready for me. They weren't as surprised as I was. It was incredibly un-psychedelic. I was able to pay attention to detail. There was one main creature, and he seemed to be behind it all, overseeing everything. The others were orderlies or dis-orderlies. They activated a sexual circuit, and I was flushed with amazing orgasmic energy. A goofy chart popped up like an X-ray in a cartoon, and a yellow illumination indicated that the corresponding system, or series of systems, were fine. They were checking my instruments, testing things. When I was coming out, I couldn't help but think 'aliens.' I am so disappointed I didn't talk to them. I was confused and in awe. I knew that they were preparing me for something. Somehow, we had a mission. They had things to show me. But they were waiting for me to acquaint myself with the environment and movement and language of this space."[25]

-Jacques Vallee, a UFO researcher, often spoke of the connections between fairies, little people, and UFO experiences, indicating that the incidents might simply all be the same thing and are shaped by the witnesses' culture.

The fact that people taking psychedelics and those who claim they were taken on board a UFO both describe seeing the same being indicates that there might be some connection between them. They could be the same beings seen from different perspectives, which would mean that reality may not be as solid as we think.

Since these entities cannot be seen, except at high doses, it supports the theory that there are various levels of reality. What is going on is that specific concentrations of psychedelics will shut down individual brain modules working together to allow the newly activated areas to open up to the reality where the entities exist.

This would be like the case of neuroanatomist Jill Bolte Taylor. She had a brain hemorrhage where she stated that at a certain point where blood was knocking neurons offline, the voice in her head shut off immediately, like pressing the mute button on the remote control, and she was thrust into a new reality where all the rules had changed.

Perhaps all dimensions exist simultaneously and occupy the same space, just at different vibrations, frequencies, or densities of energy. Dreams are a prime example. We dream at night and are in a state parallel to our normal waking state. At the same time, our body is in a bed sleeping - we are present in each simultaneously.

This would help to explain why even though serotonergic psychedelics such as DMT, LSD, mescaline, and psilocybin act as agonists at cortical 5-HT2A receptors and have a similar structure, they each will take you to a different reality.

Vibration

> *Crucially, the nature of the music experience was significantly predictive of reductions in depression one week after psilocybin, whereas general drug intensity was not.*
> **-Beckley Foundation[26]**

> *If you want to find the secrets of the universe, think in terms of energy, frequency, and vibration.*
> **-Nikola Tesla, inventor and engineer.**

Vibration is something that I experienced a great deal during my sessions. All seemed like high frequency, but some were higher frequency than others. The higher the frequency was, the smoother it seemed. Yes, it did have a texture. As common as it was for me, I did not find much on the internet of other people pointing it out. Those accounts usually talked about sounds, colors, and images. These almost didn't exist in my sessions.

In my limited understanding, there are two different ways to experience psilocybin in therapy. Stanislav Grof was a pioneer in the clinical uses of LSD back in the 1950s when he was researching and treating people with it. He is also the father of holotropic breathwork:

> *It is remarkably interesting for artists, the changes of the environment...there you get the mixture of what you see out there, and then what you are projecting. The real journey begins when you keep your eyes closed. When we do it therapeutically, we do it with eyes shades, headphones, and music. Then you just get pure messages from your unconscious. Then it becomes an extremely important investigative tool. I compared it in my early writings to the microscope and the telescope.*[27]

I used the clinical method employed by Johns Hopkins and NYU Universities. They use music and a process of attempting to go inside one's own mind. Usually, the music they use has no English lyrics to prevent activation, and therefore distraction, of the language in the left brain. It has no sudden changes in rhythm. In the early part of a session, music provides a support structure. Carefully selected music in high-dose sessions "increases the probability of increased constructive outcomes and decreases the probability of unconstructive high anxiety states."[28]

One participant in the Beckley Foundation Psilocybin study described it this way:

> *I feel the music, in large part, drove a lot of the experience. Under the influence of psilocybin, the music absolutely takes over. Normally when I hear a piece of sad music or happy music, I respond through choice... but under psilocybin, I felt almost that I had no choice but to go with the music. [...] I did feel I was being held. And it did feel like the music opened [me] up to grief, and I just was very happy for that to happen. It wasn't particularly pleasant in any way but extraordinarily powerful.[29]*

When using this process, I understood how vital the music might be in the whole process. During the height of the session, it appeared that I was no longer listening to music, but was in the music and seemed to be the music. It was a bizarre feeling that was impossible to reproduce by listening to the same music later.

Even more strange, I realized what was also described by Dr. William Richards, who worked at the psychedelic unit at Johns Hopkins. In listening to the music, which I rarely listen to, I could feel the composer's emotion as he composed it.

In a couple of sessions, I was sure that someone was messing with the music, as it fits in so well with the emotion and feeling that I was having. Either Johns Hopkins really knew something about putting music together, or there was some strange synchronicity going on.

The other possibility is that the emotion was playing off the music. The higher the dose, the more influential the music had in driving the experience. It is almost as if emotion in the physical world is only 10% active. The higher the dose, the more the insulation is taken off the emotional wires, and the more sensitive the emotion becomes. That may be where the term raw emotion comes from.

Session #5 is an example where a distracting noise was very noticeable, and when my audio recorder's button turned on, it was like an alarm clock going off next to my ear.

In thinking back on my sessions, I cannot tell you what song was playing. However, I can remember the music's tempo and intensity and how crescendos in the music would drive the emotion at that moment. This indicated to me that it is more the vibration of the music playing than what the song was or who wrote it.

The Power of Psilocybin

Analyzing the data we had found, we were not surprised to find a substantial placebo effect on depression. What surprised us was how small the drug effect was. Seventy-five percent of the improvement in the drug (SSRI) group also occurred when people were given dummy pills with no active ingredient in them... when published and unpublished data are combined, they fail to show a clinically significant advantage for antidepressant medication over inert placebo... 89% of depressed patients

are not receiving a clinically significant benefit from the antidepressants that are prescribed for them.
-Researcher Dr. Irving Kirsch Harvard Medical School

My psychiatrist diagnosed me as a Hypochondriac. I said, "Okay, can you prescribe me a placebo?"
"Not for Type-2 Hypochondriacs," he said. "Your types would just fake faking. Then we'd have a real problem."
-Brian Spellman

There is no such thing as a placebo erection.
-Steven Wright

P silocybin is a compound that has been used for almost everything under the sun. It is used for end-of-life anxiety, alcohol addiction, smoking cessation, PTSD, untreatable depression, anorexia, Alzheimer's, and the list keeps getting longer. One study of 75 participants showed that "Participants showed significant positive changes on longitudinal measures of interpersonal closeness, gratitude, life meaning/purpose, forgiveness, death transcendence, daily spiritual experiences, religious faith and coping."[30]

Some have asked if this is a panacea. Strangely, it should be to be able to deal with so many things that appear so wholly different.

One answer may lie in understanding reality. In his lectures, physicist Dr. Amit Goswami provided an expression that, if taken seriously, would help explain what is going on. He said, "It's all oollie stuff," and it's all connected. In other words, it's all consciousness, which is all one thing. Nothing can get behind consciousness.

Max Planck put it this way, "I regard consciousness as fundamental. I regard matter as derivative from consciousness. We cannot get behind consciousness. Everything that we talk about, everything that we regard as existing, postulates consciousness."

The mistake we make is to buy into the old dualistic model of matter and spirit. This old model would say that scary psychedelic drugs can create mental problems but that physical illnesses come from outside forces or bad genes. Now we see that psychedelics can cure mental issues and that physical problems can be psychosomatic.

If consciousness is primary, then matter comes from consciousness. There is no separation, and everything starts with consciousness. If it starts with consciousness, then that aspect plays a vital role in the disease's physical appearance.

As separation is synonymous with objectivity, where we can stand apart and observe what is "out there," then no separation means subjectively perceived reality. We orchestrate what we see.

It should then be no surprise that changing our thoughts will influence or cure all manner of disease. We choose instead to tell the patient they are a victim of something outside themselves that must be countered with a chemical drug, an operation, or radiation.

We already know that a placebo's power (positive efficiency effect) is being misused by the medical establishment every day. If you get healthy using a natural remedy, they say that it only worked because it is just a placebo.

There is no attempt by the medical community to explain what the placebo is, which is sometimes just as effective as anti-depressants. This makes sense as the pharmaceutical industry is only interested in making money. The money only comes by being a drug dealer of legal pharmaceuticals that must be taken for the rest of a person's life.

Guy Sapirstein and Irving Kirsch's research showed how little the SSRI effect was and how significant the placebo effect was. They found that 75% of improvements occurred when the patients were given a sugar pill (placebo) with no active ingredients, and only 25% might have been effective from the effect of the drug.

When this finding was made public and challenged, they made a Freedom of Information Act request to the FDA for all anti-depressant test results. They discovered that the drug companies had not published 27 of the 27 results in the clinical trials because they showed no benefit over taking the placebo. Only 43% of all the studies of those taking antidepressants showed statistically significant benefits over placebo. According to Kirsch, that effect would allow them to use the law term "safe and effective," but it was not clinically significant. 57% had failed to show better than placebo results. An analysis done by Kirsch and Saperstein showed that 82% of the drug response was duplicated by placebo.[31] It was the belief in the pill, and not the drug itself, that made the person better.

To explain the placebo pill, science has used what I call the naming theory. Give it a name and make it go away. Placebo is the power of the mind. Psychedelics may just be increasing the power of the placebo mind, but it results in 80% of all treatment-resistant depression or PTSD be cured. The published data on SSRI shows 20% to 30% of patients achieve complete remission.

Bruce Lipton is one of the fathers of epigenetics (control of the genes based on the environment), which is now a key area of study related to the disease. Lipton became famous for showing that a stem cell could be changed into muscle, bone, or fat cells just by changing the medium in which it was placed. He realized that consciousness could influence how the genes expressed themselves, which in turn determined the emergence of disease. We were not victims of our genes but of our perception of how the environment changes the way genes express themselves. We can therefore change the environment, our perception of it, and therefore our genes. DNA is a blueprint that cannot turn itself on and off. A gene doesn't know what it does. The contractor (mind) is the one who reads the blueprint.

"Just like a single cell," said Lipton, "the character of our lives is determined not by our genes but by our responses to the environmental signals that propel life...gene activity can change daily. If the perception in your mind is reflected in the chemistry of your body, and if your nervous system reads and interprets the environment and then controls the blood's chemistry, then you can change the fate of your cells by altering your thoughts."

Going Within

Inward is not a direction. Inward is a dimension.
-Sadhguru Jaggi

Do not feel lonely; the entire universe is inside of you.
-Rumi

I'm not looking for the light in the darkness; I'm looking for my eyes to adjust to the darkness so that I can go deeper into the darkness... we need those folks who are going to go out and encounter the entities that are in these places and spaces because they are there.
-High-dose psilocybin advocate, Kilindi Lyi.

Going within is something I did not understand until doing my first high-dose session. Going within is easier said than done. It encompasses set and setting and creating an intention. It plays on the idea that our consciousness is creating instead of believing someone outside the self influences us.

When experiencing, I realized that it had much to do with the fact that actual reality maybe something within us and not the world we see. The process of going within seems to create miraculous changes in perspective.

Quantum physics has touched on this in statements by Nobel Prize winners like Dr. John Wheeler, who said, "there is no out there out there," and "it's a participatory universe."

UFO abductees also touched on these possible inner dimensions. Many started telling stories that sounded much more like trips to matrix worlds through events that sound like near-death experiences and out-of-body experiences than trips through walls in a straight 3D environment.

Many experiences on high-dose psilocybin are quite similar to other non-chemical methods like meditation, which is a process of going within.

Many like alternative medicine advocate Deepak Chopra state that "an observer-independent reality is not testable." That is because everything eventually goes through consciousness. Similarly, John Wheeler talked about a participator reality, where we cannot be independent of what we are seeing and testing.

What happens with Psilocybin and the other psychedelics is that the observer feels like it is different. Many university tests are done lying down with a guide which would indicate that the experience is inside rather than the person traveling anywhere. It fits with Jesus's teaching that "The kingdom of heaven is within," or the Indian concept of "the pathless path."

The Female Universe

The Tao that can be told of is not the eternal Tao; The name that can be named is not the eternal name. The Nameless is the origin of Heaven and Earth; The Named is the mother of all things.

-The opening lines of Tao Te Ching

In a couple of my trips, I came across a force that seemed to represent the Universe. There was a very definite female essence to what I was dealing with in two of the three encounters.

In the physical world of nouns, the idea is that their various body parts distinguish males and females. However, in the non-local world, these physical differences are not apparent, but the sexes' impression is still there.

One example comes from people who have encounters with non-human intelligences. When the researchers ask for details of the NHI encounters, they will ask questions like, "Were you scared" or "Did they probe you" or "Was it painful."

When I question them, I usually ask, "Did the being have any clothes on?" The usual reply is no. When I ask if they saw sex organs, they usually also reply no. How then, I ask, do you know it was a male or a female. The reply is, "I just knew. I sensed it."

That was my experience. I just sensed it, but it came with absolute certainty.

As I looked at this bizarre sense, at first I thought it was just some oddity, but at one point, it seemed to make sense that it could be true. The idea would be that the universe is female, as my experience with the female I sensed had nothing to do with physical attributes.

What if, I thought, the universe is female at its core and added the male attribute to create a duality by adding negative energy, separation, and ego?

This made sense to me for the following reasons:

- The physical male component of the brain is seen as the left brain. That is where the ego (belief in separation) resides. It is where language resides, which creates the illusion of nouns and separation. The right brain sees Oneness, such as the maternal instinct of women caring for the family.

- God has always been considered the one who would involve no duality. Duality comes in with the creation of lower physical realms.

- This is confirmed by anyone who does doomscrolling every morning on their cell phone. The negative stories are almost exclusively male. Male mass murderers are killing in crowds, schools, and Jewish synagogues. (From 1982 to 2020 figures: 113 men to 3 women) There are stories of pointless disputes and fights to control countries. Wars are the ultimate symbol of separation. Bad stories are almost exclusively male-generated headlines. "Females have lower arrest rates than males for virtually all crime categories except prostitution. This is true in all countries for which data are available. It is true for all racial and ethnic groups and every historical period. In the United States, women constitute less than 20 percent of arrests for most crime categories."[32]

- Nature is generally seen as female, as in mother nature—the female runs the ant colony and the beehive. In most situations, the male is only necessary for a moment to provide sperm. When it comes to the environment, there is nothing wrong with it. It exactly knows what to do. The problem comes in the humans' minds that see the environment as an object to be tamed, used, and dominated. To me, it is the male left-brain attitudes that cause problems in female nature.

- What I was dealing with seemed much in line with what is called the attributes of the female right brain compared to the models of the male left brain:

The left side of our brain is the masculine force. It is the part of us that is assertive, logical, analytical, doing, controlling, aggressive, striving, projecting, hard, organizing, rushing, thrusting, always pushing us to survive, and has its origin in our minds.	The right side of the brain is feminine or that which is creative, delicate, intuitive, nurturing, receptive, tender, surrendering, synthesizing, integrating, soft, feeling, and the part of us that "knows" without explanation.

The Dream Connection

From the altered brainwaves and participants' reports, it's clear these people are completely immersed in their experience — it's like daydreaming only far more vivid and immersive, it's like dreaming but with your eyes open."
-Research done on DMT at the National Institute for Health Research (NIHR) Imperial Clinical Research Facility

Dreaming appears to be an essential vehicle for unconscious emotional processing and learning. By using psilocybin to enter a dreamlike state, people could deal with the stresses of trauma or depression.

-Psychiatrist Adam Winstock at the South London and Maudsley NHS Foundation Trust

This is just an idea that occurred to me after tracking my dreams and psilocybin trips.

Is it possible that the psilocybin event is just happening farther in the field but is related to dreams?

Who is setting up the dreams we have every night? It may be our spirit guides, God, or our higher self that influence our dreams and teaches us something that we need to address and work on in our lives.

That seems to be what is happening in the psilocybin trip. The difference is that while on psychedelics, these lessons are much more evident, easier to see, and we remember more of them when we come back.

The intelligence behind the psilocybin gives us what we need. The same could be said of the intelligence behind dreams. If we casually jump into a psilocybin experience or resist what is happening during it, it can quickly turn into a bad trip. Perhaps the same principle applies in dreams, but we do not see the connection because it is more nebulous.

A critical question remains – who is in charge of the events in a dream or a mushroom journey? I would not be surprised if they were closely related.

Ego Death- The Premortem Death

I got to see what really goes on. I get spiritual dimensions every time I go out, whether it is 200mg or 500 mg because I have broken that wall (ego) down. What used to be a real dramatic crumbling of the ego and all this stuff. Now I find that I make that transition only by finding out that I have made it. I go, "I am over here now, and there is God, and whatever else." That is because it is about the work for me – the work on the psychological stuff. God shows up, and it's like, Hey, how's it going?
-Kara from the Portland Psychedelic Society

E go death is one of the most important lessons that is learned during a high-dose psilocybin experience. On a neurological level, the default mode network (DMN) is being shut down. It is safe to say that all research on psychedelic states agrees with this notion.

The DMN is the resting wakefulness state of the brain where it is focused on the outside world. It is made up of:

A cortically defined set of network nodes. Consisting of distinct regions/nodes distributed across the ventromedial and lateral prefrontal, posteromedial, and inferior parietal, as well as the lateral and medial temporal cortex, the DMN is considered a backbone of cortical integration...Seed-based functional connectivity studies further demonstrate additional DMN-specific connectivity to several subcortical structures, including the amygdala and striatum.33

Researchers like Dennis McKenna describe the network as the brain area that creates the "reality hallucination." This consists of the ego, where we believe we are an individual that is separate from all that is around us. McKenna states that:

It is a set of processing tools that takes information in from the external world, and a lot of what the brain does is filter things out. It is not so much a gateway for information. It is a very tight valve that makes sure only certain things get through – the important things to your immediate survival. The associated and processing parts of the cortex will relate to memories that are learned patterns, learned things that have happened to you, or your anticipation of the future. The DMN interprets your direct experience in terms of what it already knows, like patterns that it already knows. Nothing is ever novel...the ego part is this narration of the show that makes up your reality hallucination.34

High-dose psychedelics temporarily disable the DMN. It takes it off-line. The ego and the little voice in your head that always narrates is shut off or quietened. This opens the filter and allows other parts of reality to be seen. When this false ego in the left brain is calmed, the real observer that watches the ego comes to the forefront.

"What psychedelics do," said McKenna:

Is bring the background, and they suppress what is always in our background. That is a precious thing because a lot is going on in the background that we are conditioned never to notice. After all, we think they are not important. They are important. You take the DMN off-line, and you can open yourself up to all these other things that you never pay attention to. You realize, wow, I am missing a lot...these are important aspects of reality that I never noticed before...you realize that these things are more important than what your ego and DMN forces you to look at all the time.

There are other ways to disable the DMN, such as meditation, near-death experience, and when blood floods the DMN circuit. Jill Bolte Taylor best described this in her book, *A Stroke of Insight*, about her left-brain hemorrhage that took this circuit offline for seven weeks.

I had tried meditation, hypnosis, and lucid dreaming. I have never had a near-death experience, so it was not until I used the modality of psilocybin that I could shut down my DMN.

Like everyone who has reported the experience, I realized that I am the person behind the little voice, not the voice in my head. Like many others taking psilocybin, I felt I was connected to everything around me and saw that separation is an illusion that the DMN creates.

When the experience is over, the DMN network comes back online. Still, as most people report, it is like the brain-computer has to be defragged and rewired, and possibly many illnesses like addiction, PTSD, depression, and anxiety can then be healed.

Fear

I think fear is in relationship to left-brain thinking...From the moment you have the thought that there's a threat and that circuit of fear gets triggered, it will stimulate the emotional circuitry related to it, which is the fight or flight reaction.
-Dr. Jill Bolte Taylor

When you do take larger doses, you do run the risk of unearthing some genuinely horrifying, painful stuff. Although we will slay the dragon of the myth, there still are some dragons, but they are your dragons. Since 1986 I have done 150 high dose LSD and 150-morning glory high dose sessions, and I have never met anything evil.
-Kara, the founder of Vancouver Washington Psychedelic Shamanism meetup group

Fear is a creation of our left-brain circuitry. It is also a big part of any discussion about psilocybin. People will talk about the fear of taking too much of the drug, fear of not being ready, fear of things that happen during the experience, and fear of long-lasting adverse effects from the mushrooms themselves.

Harvard neuroanatomist Jill Bolte Taylor discussed fear concerning a left-brain stroke that knocked out her left-brain functions for seven weeks. She spoke of the value of the experience where she had "gotten as much out of this experience of losing my left mind as I have in my entire academic career."[35] In talking about her experience, she reminded people that fear is "false evidence appearing real."

In an interview with Forbes magazine, Taylor stated that once the blood from the bleeding flooded the left brain, it went offline "I had zero fear. I was there in blissful euphoria in the right brain."[36] The fear disappeared and did not reappear until the left-brain came back online.

I had a lot of fear making the first trip and going into the high dose 4th session. Once I was in the session four experience, I looked back and realized that I had worried about nothing. It seemed so stupid.

Johns Hopkins University and other labs do warn about the bad trip, which they call negative aspects. The highest dose they gave was 30mg/70kg, which led to the following results:

> *Researchers noted that the reported positive effects increased as higher doses were given, but also that there was a sharp increase in the negative aspects at the very highest dose. At the highest dose (30 mg/70 kg, p.o. - meaning "per oral" or by mouth), 78 percent of the volunteers were reporting one of the top five most spiritually significant happenings of their lives, but those suffering anxiety, stress, and fear episodes increased by six times so that around a third of those participating in the study showed signs of psychological struggle.*[37]

Lower doses had fewer negative aspects, and the scientists concluded that dosage was crucial in both positive and negative effects. This would make sense that the higher dosages would move you further from the physical consciousness, and more repressed emotions would be exposed:

> *By contrast, only one of the volunteers receiving the second-highest dose (20mg/70 kg, p.o.) reported having negative issues, and all benefited from positive experiences, although with less intensity than at the highest dose.*[38]

What has always bothered me about this generalization is why I had no negative experiences. I don't think I have had a life devoid of repressed guilt, shame, or negative experiences.

Perhaps it is the ego in the left brain that creates fear. It is always trying to create fear scenarios to keep us safe. It also makes those false scenarios because it tends to see things in a negative light.

We know that fear does not exist without the left brain based on Jill Bolte Taylor's testimony.

Another way of putting one's experience into perspective is to understand what Joseph Campbell refers to as the "Hero's Journey." The journey begins with the hero leaving his home, going to a strange and unknown place, encountering challenges and temptations, and returning home forever transformed. Carl Jung's concept of the Shadow is also helpful to a further understanding of what has transpired. The shadow is the dark side of our personality. It is that part of ourselves that we do not want to acknowledge and keep hidden from the world

The Bad Trip

Until you make the unconscious conscious, it will direct your life, and you will call it fate.
-Carl Jung

Turning toward rather than away from one's experience is a good lesson for life in general and is also relevant to the psychedelic experience.
-Sara Gael, harm reduction officer at the Zendo Project

We [Western societies] have no tradition of shamanism. We have no tradition of journeying into these mental worlds. We are terrified of madness.
-Terence McKenna

The bad trip has been a card that gets played over and over in many conversations surrounding psychedelics. Drama queens may wish to center on this aspect of the experience as it contains the excitement they seek in life.

Many, or even most scientists who work on psychedelics, have brought it up at some point. This may center around them viewing themselves as the "priestly class" who want to control what happens. People believe that bad trips will befall them if they do not have their hands held by those who believe they have superior information about what is going on.

Politicians are the bad trip's biggest promoters because they see their role as the voting sheep's guardians. They see themselves as lawmakers who make people happy and protect them from bad things like psychedelics.

Most politicians are not against drugs per se. They favor certain drugs like alcohol, caffeine, and nicotine that keep their citizens working and happy and provide patients for their private hospitals that treat the ill effects of the "legal" drugs.

Politicians are also sympathetic to drug companies that make the drugs. They help fuel their political campaigns that require ever-increasing funding for their election and re-election. Every politician knows not to bite the hand that feeds them and employs their constituents.

Politicians are also sympathetic to legal drugs that provide tax dollars to pay for public programs like roads and bridges. The best example of this is the conservative provincial government that runs Manitoba, where I live.

When Prime Minister Justin Trudeau pushed through his legislation to legalize cannabis, the conservatives did everything in their power to stop it. In 2017, when they realized they probably couldn't stop it, they agreed but insisted there would be no allocation for homegrown cannabis. (which naturally brings in no tax dollars).

When it was finally legalized, the Conservative government controlled it all through government-run stores, and the tax dollars are now plentiful.

One story that clearly shows legality has nothing to do with the safety of the drug but rather the political party in and who controls the drug's sales came in 2020 during the COVID-19 situation. There was a complete shutdown in April, including hairdressers, restaurants, bars, any store that didn't sell food, churches, and movie theatres, except for "essential services." Essential services, of course, included liquor and cannabis stores. Cannabis had gone from the devil's weed to an essential service in a few short years.

Lastly, some of the "bad trip" belief comes from the propaganda put out by the Nixon administration. Their move to make psychedelics illegal came from an effort to arrest and silence the people who did not vote for them. John Ehrlichman, who acted as Richard Nixon's counsel and Assistant to the President for Domestic Affairs, stated:

> *You understand what I'm saying? We knew we couldn't make it illegal to be either against the war or black, but by getting the public to associate the hippies with marijuana and blacks with heroin. And then criminalizing both heavily, we could disrupt those communities. We could arrest their leaders. Raid their homes, break up their meetings, and vilify them night after night on the evening news. Did we know we were lying about the drugs? Of course, we did.*

Ralph Metzner, a psychologist, writer, and researcher who participated in psychedelic research at Harvard

University in the early 1960s with Timothy Leary and Richard Alpert, described the day he learned that the bad psychedelic trip was merely the creation of his own consciousness.

During a Harvard research project where prisoners and researchers were being dosed, Metzner recalled one bad trip that he had:

> *There were no bad trips. There were bad trips in terms of some parts of the trips that were horrendous. Some of my experiences were horrendous – hell visions. I remember these horrendous hell visions, and then one time I was lying on the bed, and I was going through this macabre hell thing like Stan Grof would say BPM2. Then I would open my eyes, and there would be a group of guys, some of the cons, and some of the students quietly sitting smoking with the afternoon light coming in. There were extreme peacefulness and serenity. I realized, "Oh my God. That whole hell was in my head. There was no hell. It was all in my head. It was all gone once I opened my eyes. That was profound."*[39]

After all of my experiences, I was left with the impression that it is fear and not dosage level that is a critical factor in whether you have a good or bad trip. If someone goes in with a high dosage and no fear, they will not be affected. However, if they go in with a low dosage and a lot of fear, they may be in for a rough ride.

Another psilocybin researcher once said, "There are no bad trips. If you have one, you are just learning at a rate you are unaccustomed to." According to Johns Hopkins, the higher the dose, the greater the chance that there will be an element of a so-called "bad trip."

As the dosage increases, the emotion within the experience increases, and so do the lessons that are being presented. Psilocybin is weird because people always warn about the bad trip, and a lot of energy is used up by researchers trying to avoid it. Yet, many of the same people express praise at the ayahuasca experience.

Anyone who has read about ayahuasca encounters will hear horror stories about the intensity of the experience, the vomiting, diarrhea, and how mother ayahuasca killed them numerous times during the session.

The musician Sting from the band The Police described his encounter with ayahuasca this way:

> *I took it, went to my hammock, and tied the seatbelt on. I was destroyed. I just simply didn't exist. I basically crawled to the shaman and said, please put me back together again.*

In the ayahuasca experience, deeply held trauma may surface, and those who have no awareness of the nature of such experiences can find it overwhelming. Those who travel to places like Peru to participate in ceremonies are aware of these risks and know they must go through them.

Strangely, there seems to be a belief that people should be sheltered from encountering these unconsciously held traumas when taking psychedelics like psilocybin, LSD, and DMT. It is thought that traumatic experiences during trips should be eliminated because they are too scary. Candy trips only, please! don't put these poor people through something bad. But this exactly is what must be done. It is almost as if dealing with these difficult experiences has been replaced by people only wanting to have a good time.

Stanislav Grof has talked about "bad trips" for decades. Grof worked with LSD therapies back in the 1950s in Europe and has guided over 4,500 LSD sessions. He also developed holotropic breathwork, a breathing technique that can produce the same visions and ego death experienced during a psychedelic trip.

Grof, too, does not go along with the efforts to avoid the bad trip and focuses on taking psychedelics for trauma integration. He goes as far as to suggest that if someone has a bad trip, the worst thing you can do is try and bring them out. This is what he told interviewer Tim Ferris:

> *I very early discovered that if you have a bad trip, there's no good way of terminating it. The worst thing that you can do is what's done routinely, which is calm with tranquilizers. When you give tranquilizers to people who are on a bad trip and then keep them on maintained dosages, this prevents any kind of resolution. If somebody has a bad trip, that means that they are dealing with a difficult aspect of their unconscious. And when it's coming up, it's coming up for healing. It's not just that the drug created this horrible experience. So, the way you do it, you have to tell people that you are in an LSD session, "This is a time-limited thing. I'm going to be here."*
>
> *And then, when something remains unresolved, you do some bodywork and some emotional work to*

bring it to a good closure. People can benefit from these bad trips. So, I realized very early that when people had difficult experiences, the last thing I would do is to combine with tranquilizers. And so, I saw many of the situations where people experienced what they would be hospitalized for in the psychedelic session. And if we stayed with it, it actually was a major healing, major transformation.[40]

Bringing fear into the psychedelic experience leads people to feel like victims. When afraid, they will try and fight back or avoid what lesson is being presented to them. That is wholly opposed to the idea that I was taught in Session #5, that one must surrender.

It is for this reason that most research studies use guides. A guide's role is to be by your side and help you counter the fear that arises when there are heightened emotions. The guide takes the person's hand and tells them it is ok, and that everything is alright.

Even Terence McKenna used this process. He would take his 5-gram hero dose alone in a dark room. He would have a bell that he would ring if fear set in. That instructed someone in the next room to stick their head in the room and say everything is alright, and then they would leave. Terrance would continue with the session.

The "bad trip" idea began in the 1960s. Much of what was said was not true, and the stigma has carried on to the present day. Some of the bad reports that scared people were just words said out of ignorance, preventing people from trying whatever psychedelic it is.

An example is a story about 5-MeO-DMT told by Michael Pollan to 2.3 million people who heard the interview. Pollan wrote a book on his psychedelic research that the New York Times identified as a #1 bestseller and one of the 10 top books of 2018. Pollan told Rogan that his 5-MeO-DMT experience was terrible, so Rogan asked him what happened as his own experience had been positive.

Pollan stated that he had used the secretion from a toad's venom glands, dried, and smoked. He took one hit and recalled a horrible experience with no real information given to him during the trip:

> *You are shot out of a cannon, and there is no leadup. There is no warmup. I felt that I was strapped to the outside of a rocket, going through space and clouds. The g-forces were pulling down my cheeks. It was just this mental storm with nothing to orient myself. There was no space. There was no time. There was no self. It was just punishing with this unbelievable roar in my ears...what happened to me is I had the storm...it was just this incoherent energy...it was horrible. It was terrifying. I thought I was dying...an experienced Psychonaut told me that I didn't have enough.*[41]

"That is what I was going to tell you as well," said Rogan. Rogan claimed his experience was wonderful, and he brought back lots of information, mostly about himself.

They talked back and forth, and it became evident that Pollan had only inhaled once when the clear procedure is that you only have about 9 seconds and need to get in three tokes.

"I guess I did something wrong," said Pollan.

He did do something wrong. It is evident that the guide he used did not know, or did not correctly show Pollan what to do, didn't count down the 9 seconds, or worse, didn't know himself what he was administering and charging for.

Sadly, that misconstrued "bad trip" story stays in a #1 best-selling book for everyone to read.

Finally, I would say that a bad trip comes from facing the shadow figures inside our consciousness placed in our experience by our higher self to deal with. Dr. David Nutt made a critical point, a Professor of Neuropsychopharmacology at Imperial College London and the director of the Neuropsychopharmacology Unit in the Division of Brain Sciences. He pointed out that all the subjects with resistant depression in his research study had bad psilocybin trips because they were working out, or remodeling, the brain circuits that were causing the depression:

> *Some people take recreational trips, and they have bad trips, yet they say, 'I feel different, and I see the world more logically,' so even a bad trip can be beneficial. Usually, they don't want another one, but they can have benefit. The reality is that in our depression study, people do not have good trips. A psilocybin trip lasts 4- 5 hours, and all of them are going somewhere that is dark and unpleasant. It is often stated that they repressed for decades. That allows them to get into the origins of their depression to try and find the causation or one of the elements of their depression. These are not pleasurable. These people are not having ecstasy. These people are having agony.*[42]

The testimony of Jodie Long backs up Nutt's assessment that bad trips result from some issue that needs to be addressed. She is in charge of the roughly 4,800 near-death experiences posted on the Near-Death Experience Research Foundation (NDERF) website. She talked about negative NDEs that are undergone about 10% of the time. Long said, "I think that when people have these (negative experiences), you are normally going to see people that need to wake up, or they need to change their direction. Otherwise, they are not going to the most spiritual life out of their body that they need to get out of this incarnation."[43]

Someone in the Room

This was something that I experienced in Session #6. It was a situation that startled me both times, one worse than the other.

Because I had a blindfold on and music going in my headset, the physical world around me was completely cut off.

When the incidents happened, it can be likened to being in a daydream and someone coming up to see if you are okay. They do not say or do anything, and at a point, you suddenly realize they are standing there looking at you. It is quite alarming.

In Session #6, I felt like someone was standing on my right, just beside the bed, between me and my computer. The second incident was much more frightening because I got the feeling that this person had turned on my light.

Quickly pulling up the blindfold revealed an utterly dark room both times with no one being there. I was still left shaking over the very distinct feeling someone had been there.

After I had finished Session #8, a podcast about psychedelics advised using meditation to revisit the experiences and integrate them. I decided to try this. What I did was sit blindfolded in front of the computer, listen to choral music, and meditate.

Unlike the psilocybin sessions where you remain awake, I drifted off asleep while sitting up. Suddenly, I had the sense of someone beside me on my right side. I bolted up and looked from under the blindfold. It was dark, and there was no one there. There may have been no one there both times, but the feeling was as real as anything I have experienced in the 3D hallucinatory reality.

No self

I believe that the more time we spend choosing to run the deep inner-peace circuitry of our right hemispheres, the more peace we will project into the world, and the more peaceful our planet will be.
-Neuroanatomist Jill Bolte Taylor

If the ego has an address, it is in the default mode network.
-Michael Pollan

So, ego should be a controlled substance?

-Steven Colbert

This section may be the most important in the whole book. Is there a *self* that walks around in life? Is there a subject-object split where there is an individual and then independent objects surrounding him or her?

The more puzzle pieces we gather about reality, the more it appears that there may just be consciousness, and the self is an illusion created to have this experience. As the theory goes, everything that happens in the 3D world is nothing more than an event in consciousness. If this is true, then it is time to rethink everything.

This view of reality supports the many reports that people who have made the psilocybin trip strongly believe that the self is an illusion created in the left brain. When those cells in that part of the brain are taken off-line, the self disappears simultaneously as the conscious awareness is maintained. The person then becomes aware of the new concept that they are one with everything around them. The former worldview is now just a habitual behavior like smoking or cocaine addiction that is no longer needed.

The neurological discussions of what is going on describe the quieting of the Default Mode Network (DMN), which is known as the "orchestrator of the self." As stated before, this quieting can also be done with non-drug processes such as holotropic breathwork and meditation.

Jill Bolte Taylor worked in the brain lab at Harvard University on severe mental illnesses. She experienced a left-brain hemorrhage in September 1996 in her apartment. Here she discusses how that led to the dissolution of the ego and the little voice that goes along with it:

> *And at that moment, my left hemisphere brain chatter went totally silent. Just like someone took a remote control and pushed the mute button. Total silence. And at first, I was shocked to find myself inside of a silent mind. But then I was immediately captivated by the magnificence of the energy around me. And because I could no longer identify the boundaries of my body, I felt enormous and expansive. I felt at one with all the energy that was.[44]*

What I experienced and what many others have reported on psilocybin was described by Taylor in her traumatic stroke experience:

> *What I gained was this incredible knowingness of deep inner peace and excitement of realizing everything was interconnected, and I lost the boundary of my body, so I felt that I was enormous as big as the universe because I no longer defined that this was where I began and this was where I ended more.[45]*

Beta brainwaves dominate our normal waking state of consciousness when our attention is directed towards cognitive tasks and the outside world. Beta is the 'fast' activity present when one is alert, attentive, engaged in problem-solving, judgment, decision making, or focused mental activity.

Brain Chemistry

It goes back to the division of the mind and the body, or the brain and the mind and the body, or the soul; there's no division.
-Jill Bolte Taylor

Human beings will do just about anything to resolve contradictions between our deeply held beliefs about the world and the reality of the world itself. Cognitive dissonance is so unpleasant, so disordering and catastrophic for the ego that no amount of absurd, tortured reasoning is worse than reality contradicting a deeply held belief.
-Daily Beast reporter Jay Michaelson talks about "dead-enders."

Who directs the movement of blood in the brain? Who directs the dream? Who directs the trip?

Many materialists hold tightly to the belief that the psilocybin experience is nothing but brain chemistry. This idea will soon go by the wayside like the rational, analytical thinkers of the 15th century who believed the Earth was flat.

Scientists claim they understand reality then change their minds and claim to have proven a different reality all time time. This is all due to a small bundle of neurons that constitute the left-brain interpreter (LBI). The LBI is a crucial component of the rational, analytical mind and is involved in many theories we then take as proof.

The left brain interpreter takes data from all the five senses, and its job is to come up with an explanation when what is given in terms of data becomes inconsistent. The main discovery that was made about the reason that the Interpreter believes is that:

1) The Interpreter guesses and will never say "I don't know," which would be the truthful reply.

2) The guess that it comes up with is almost always wrong. Michael Gazzaniga, a psychology professor at the University in California, called this *the narrative fallacy.*

3) It believes the nonsense it has put out and could easily pass a lie detector

4) Once the Interpreter makes a guess, it will never back off and will fight to the death to defend the fact it was right.

This is where skepticism comes from. Skeptics rarely read the data before they make their conclusions. Ufologist Stanton Friedman described it this way after debating skeptics about UFOs for 61 years, "Don't bother me with the evidence. My mind is already made up." *Skeptics will make up an instant explanation for things they don't understand, like the paranormal. The LBI jumps in to try to explain the unexplainable. Really good skeptics are just people whose LBI works super fast.* Once they provide a counter explanation to make the old-world view consistent, they will continue to double down and will never back off the explanation they offered.

Gazzaniga's work showed that the Interpreter could be manipulated and tricked. He calls it "hijacking," — and when the Interpreter is hijacked, it makes pretty bad decisions and generates strange explanations.

Much of the argument about psilocybin merely being brain chemistry has been created by the Interpreter guessing why these altered states happen.

The fact that I had entirely different experiences each time would negate the idea that the incident was being caused only by chemicals lighting up neurons. If that were the only factor, the experience should have been the same every time because the same brain modules would have been affected by the chemicals.

The default mode network is indeed being shut down during the psilocybin event, but who is shutting it down? The DMN will be getting less blood, but who is regulating the flow of blood? Does the brain have a brain that moves blood around?

The fact that the left-brain DMN is turned off could be explained by the idea that the DMN creates noise that hides the signal. When it is shut down, the awareness can pick up the higher vibrating reality.

In a study led by neuroscientist Robin Carhart-Harris, head of psychedelic research in the brain sciences division of the Imperial College of London medical school, they found that when "the DMN was inactive, an alternate network of consciousness seemed to arise."[46] Who then is orchestrating the shutting down of one series of modules and activating a second?

A prime example of this would be the experience of Jill Bolte Taylor. She had a left-brain hemorrhage and described a state of consciousness with many parallels to the psychedelic experience. With the left brain out of the way, Taylor explained the role of the right brain:

> *Our right human hemisphere is all about this present moment. It's all about, 'right here, right now.' Our right hemisphere thinks in pictures, and it learns kinesthetically through the movement of our bodies. Information, in the form of energy, streams in simultaneously through all of our sensory systems, and then it explodes into this enormous collage of what this present moment looks like, what this present moment smells like and tastes like, what it feels like and what it sounds like. I am an energy being connected to the energy all around me through the consciousness of my right hemisphere.*
>
> *We are energy beings connected to one another through the consciousness of our right hemispheres as one human family. And right here, right now, we are brothers and sisters on this planet, here to make the world a better place. And at this moment, we are perfect. We are whole, and we are beautiful... I felt enormous and expansive. I felt at one with all the energy that was, and it was beautiful there.*

There is, of course, no reductionist, materialistic model that would explain how this could happen. Reductionist science runs one neuron, one behavior, but that is like listening to one instrument in an orchestra and calling it music. The truth is that all the instruments and a conductor make up the orchestra that makes the music.

This problem becomes more problematic for material neurologists when we look at what Michael Gazzaniga, the father of cognitive neuroscience, stated. He asserts that the brain consists of "Small local circuits, made of an interconnected group of neurons, are created to perform specific processing jobs and become automatic." These work together as a confederation of "potentially millions" of independent modules working together.

How then do they work together? How do potentially millions of modules change what they are doing to act in a completely different way when psilocybin is introduced? Who reroutes the blood if the modules are independent? Who shuts off some modules and turns on others?

It would appear that they all work together and know what to do in the same way a bee will change its role when a hive is damaged. It will begin a rebuilding task instead of collecting pollen even though it has never built anything and has no training. It is the same principle that if a part of the brain is injured, other brain parts will change function and perform the damaged section's task. Another example of this process is the body's ability to replace 200 different cells that make up the human body. One million cells a second die in the human body and are replaced instantly. Who oversees this process? Would it be the brain that comprises millions of independent modules with no visible material organizer?

Our brain has often been referred to as a computer. The problem with this analogy is that the materialists leave out part of the computer story.

You can get the most powerful computer in the world, or you can string 15 billion together as we now have as part of the internet. But, the fact is, nothing will happen without consciousness.

How do people think the computer got built? Did it just make itself? It was created by consciousness or a whole series of conscious minds. Many of the ideas that led to the development of the computer occurred when the creators were on LSD.

Who sets up the electrical system needed for the computer? A consciousness. The computer did not build itself.

Who wires all the computers into a network? Once again, that requires a consciousness and not a computer.

Now we can wire 15 billion computers with electricity and turn the whole system on, and nothing will happen. Nothing happens because you need a consciousness to program the software that tells the computer what to do. Most importantly, you need consciousness to upload all the information, stories, and data that make up the internet.

Without consciousness doing all this, NOTHING happens. NOTHING! There is no computer, internet, or information until a human consciousness sits down and builds the system.

This commonsense understanding has been known for years and is known as "the ghost in the machine." Materialists like to talk about the machine like a whistle past the graveyard when dealing with the ghost in the machine that makes the whole thing work.

So, what comes first? The computer or the consciousness? The consciousness is primary. There is no computer without a consciousness to create it. The brain is like a computer, and like the computer has a consciousness that builds, programs, and powers it.

The brain chemistry belief really starts to fall on hard times when we look at the simple fact that the mystical states produced by psilocybin can be produced without any chemical at all. These modalities would include:

- Holotropic breathwork
- Neurofeedback training
- Mediation
- Near-death experience
- Daydreaming

These examples will produce the same states of consciousness, turn on the specific brain modules, and shut down things like the default mode network. No chemicals are needed at all. All you need is consciousness, which proves it can change and control brain function.

The Fireworks

No phenomenon is a physical phenomenon until it is an observed phenomenon.

-John Wheeler

My brain is only a receiver; in the Universe, there is a core from which we obtain knowledge, strength, and inspiration. I have not penetrated into the secrets of this core, but I know that it exists.

-Nikola Tesla

I t is now known that when a person has a psychedelic experience, what happens in the brain is not what the materialistic neurological dogma would predict.

This research was conducted by the Beckley Foundation where they used fMRIs to track "cerebral blood flow (CBF) and blood-oxygen-level-dependent (BOLD) resting-state functional connectivity (RSFC) measured with functional magnetic resonance imaging (fMRI) before and after treatment with psilocybin (serotonin agonist) for treatment-resistant depression (TRD)."[47]

Amanda Fielding, the Director at Beckley, expected an abundance of activity in the brain because of the intensity of reported psychedelic experiences. Instead, she declared:

We found that comparable SIBO psilocybin decreases blood flow and activities, particularly to a network of highly interconnected brain beauties known as a default mode network (DMN); all the data showed reductions in one flow and neural activity to this important network and the degree of the reduction correlated with the subjective effects of the psychedelic experience. [48]

In street language, this means that psilocybin does not work by ramping up the brain's activity as the Beckley-funded research expected. Instead, it reduces it. Whole-brain activity drops, particularly in specific regions densely connected to the brain's sensory areas. Psilocybin reduces activity in these nodes and severs their connection to other brain areas, allowing the senses to run free.

Indeed, Huxley and Blake had predicted a key finding of modern neuroscience; many of the human brain's highest achievements involve preventing actions instead of initiating them and sifting out useless information rather than collecting and presenting it for conscious consideration. Aldous Huxley, in his book *Doors of Perception*, 70 years ago, predicted that the brain works as a reducing valve for an experience that may be occurring elsewhere:

> *Each person is at each moment capable of remembering all that has ever happened to him and of perceiving everything that is happening everywhere in the universe. The function of the brain and nervous system is to protect us from being overwhelmed and confused by this mass of largely useless and irrelevant knowledge by shutting out most of what we should otherwise perceive or remember at any moment and leaving only that very small and special selection which is likely to be practically useful.*[49]

The point is that fireworks are going on during a psilocybin experience; much more action is occurring than in conscious experience. Reality shows that the fireworks are not being fired off in the brain. It must be happening elsewhere.

If it were so, the fMRI would pick it up. It did not, and this was Imperial College London research that has been duplicated repeatedly.

Neurologists will still maintain that it is all brain chemistry and that, somehow, we are not picking up brain activity from the vast amounts of experiences being reported. There is a straightforward reply to this idea to perpetuate the religious dogma about brain activity. Carl Sagan said, "extraordinary claims require extraordinary evidence." If the fireworks are happening in the brain, it is up to the neurologists to provide the evidence. If they cannot, they are promoting pseudoscience.

This is the same dilemma that neurology has fallen into with near-death experiences. People report that their experience was more real during their NDEs, while their brains had flatlined than in the real world. As in the psychedelic observation, there is activity reported with no brain activity being recorded.

That has led to questionable neurological theories about deep brain structures in the still active, flat-lined brain. These theories enable them to make mindless claims that the flatlined brain sees events when the eyes are closed or taped shut, as they are, while in the operating room. So the person can't see anything. The flatlined brain by virtue of its own title, is nonfunctional. Scientists want there to be a logical explanation for the fact that it sees, so it must be chemicals causing the brain to fire that cause it. But there are no chemicals, so this is a made-up explanation to explain an unknown situation. Indeed, this destroys the very paradigm they were taught when young. It is simply not logical.

Illusion: Knowing Vs. Believing

What if you slept, and what if in your sleep you dreamed? And what if in your dream you went to heaven, and there plucked a strange and beautiful flower. And what if when you awoke, you had that flower in your hand. Ah, what then?
-Samuel Taylor Coleridge, philosopher

I n my review of various discussions about psilocybin, I often hear the counter explanation that the psilocybin state is just an illusion. In this defrocking of the psilocybin experience, the basic idea is that 'I know, and the psilocybin trippers are just believing.' Their anecdotal accounts are nothing but false misconceptions that cannot be reproduced under controlled conditions. The argument fails under the following evidence:

- What on earth is an illusion? If the truth is told, it is just something outside the average human experience that the skeptical mind wants to discount. The rule, therefore, is to give it a name and make it go away.

- Consciousness is a challenging problem that has no answer. All we can know for sure is that we are aware. To assume my waking consciousness is more valid than a psilocybin experience is simply the ego talking. How does one prove that their consciousness is any more real, or anything more than a self-deluding illusion?

- The high-dose psilocybin experience is reproducible. The testimonials reporting on the experience are just as valid as testimonials received in the research done on pain killers and anti-depressants.

- Those coming back from breakthrough psychedelic experiences will describe that the experience was more real than the real world. Therefore, there is a good chance that 3D awareness is an illusion.

Time

This is just a guess based on what I experienced. When in an altered psychedelic state, people often describe that time and space no longer exist as we know them. People in the DMT state will, for example, express their ten-minute trip, stating that they were virtually gone 1,000 or more years inside the other reality. This effect brings us back to an account from 1913, where mescaline intoxication made a person feel like "the immediate future was rushing on at chaotic speed, and the time was boundless."[50]

I experienced two different states of time during my sessions. After the psilocybin had fully taken effect, there was no concept of time and space. When waiting for the psilocybin to take effect, or when coming out of the experience, however, I did have a sense of time.

Also, the time effect seemed to tie into the other feelings, such as emotion and Oneness with the music. The higher the dosage, the more time seemed to disappear.

Similarly, physicists like Einstein stated that time was an illusion. Donald Hoffman, a cognitive scientist, says there is no time or space or material matter. He added that not believing this does not change the reality.

You don't have to believe in the truth to make the truth do what you need it to do. Whatever the truth is, it's not about space-time and physical objects. That means that our perception of physical causality, which states that 'I'm moving this paper,' is a useful fiction, but it's just fiction. No physical thing has real causal powers. Clean prediction - no physical object has a definite value of any dynamical physical property like position momentum and spin when one does not observe it.[51]

Oneness and Love

I think we are beginning to suspect that man is not a tiny cog that doesn't really make much difference to the running of the huge machine but rather that there is a much more intimate tie between man and the universe than we heretofore suspected.
-John Wheeler

Learn how to see. Realize that everything connects to everything else.

— Leonardo DaVinci

Your brain is an orchestra, and each neuron is an instrument. An orchestra is an ensemble of instruments, including string, brass, woodwind, and percussion sections. Traditionally, neuroscience has focused on individual neurons. Traditionally, neuroscience has just listened to the percussion section.
-Kimberlee D'Ardenne Ph.D.

The Oneness concept is hard to explain to most people who have not experienced it, as they are imbued with a Darwinian religious faith that sees everything as random. We live in a world of survival of the fittest. This involves separate entities struggling to rape, pillage, kill, and steal. These actions lead to better performance for some, eliminating the unfit, more production, and lower prices in our society. People who have not had the Oneness experience will generally write it off as an illusion or as the brain seeing a pattern that is not there in the meaningless noise of the universe.

Neurologists will write off the Oneness experience as merely the default mode network, or DMN (which creates the illusion of separation, ego, and sense of self) being shut down. Oneness is described in all breakthrough hallucinogenic experiences, but it is not a state reserved only for psychedelics.

Engineer Dr. Edgar Mitchell experienced this on his return to the Earth. The experience led to him forming the Institute for Noetic Studies to explain what the experience means for the ultimate understanding of our reality. His non-drug experience shows convincingly that the Oneness effect may have nothing to do with physiological changes. Mitchell wrote:

> *Instead of an intellectual search, there was suddenly a very deep gut feeling that something was different. It occurred when looking at Earth and seeing this blue-and-white planet floating there, and knowing it was orbiting the Sun, seeing that Sun, seeing it set in the background of the very deep black and velvety cosmos, seeing - rather, knowing for sure - that there was a purposefulness of flow, of energy, of time, of space in the cosmos - that it was beyond man's rational ability to understand, that suddenly there was a nonrational way of understanding that had been beyond my previous experience.*
>
> *There seems to be more to the universe than a random, chaotic, purposeless movement of a collection of molecular particles.*
>
> *On the return trip home, gazing through 240,000 miles of space toward the stars and the planet from which I had come, I suddenly experienced the universe as intelligent, loving, harmonious.*[52]

Another group that has started to awaken to the Oneness concept, and that separation is an illusion, is theoretical physics. Almost 100 years ago, Erwin Schrödinger made the pronouncement that "The total number of minds in the universe is one. In fact, consciousness is a singularity phasing within all beings", and "consciousness cannot be accounted for in physical terms. For consciousness is utterly fundamental. It cannot be accounted for in terms of anything else".

David Bohm, who was Einstein's successor at Princeton University, echoed Schrödinger, saying, "Deep down, the consciousness of mankind is one mind."

This one mind is made up of all the minds of humanity. These work like an orchestra rather than the old analogy of a computer. All the modules are like instruments playing as one in the creation of the music. The Force keeps the modules working together and feels deep regret when one instrument is unhappy with the group's harmony and leaves to play his own tune. The modules in the brain are independent, but they also all work together. They work as one. The brain works as one unique thing.

The feeling of Oneness implies a lot more in the psilocybin state because the connection seems extremely obvious. One study done at Johns Hopkins University showed that "two-thirds of the group reported having a 'full mystical experience,' characterized by a feeling of 'Oneness' with the universe."

What also helps the Oneness understanding is heightened emotions. Instead of being independent of the pain around the world, a person is allowed to experience the pain they caused others. This is achieved by the experience of stripping off all the insulation from your emotional wires.

People can do a compassion meditation of Earth and say they sat and felt the pain of those suffering. The low emotional state, and separation from those suffering, makes the exercise mostly an intellectual exercise. In the psilocybin state, you are experiencing the grief as if it were happening to you with full, raw emotions attached. An analogy would be reading the obituaries in the Saturday paper and mourning the deaths compared to being each of those people as they suffered and died.

People doing very high-dose psilocybin sessions often report entering a state of hell, where they are forced to feel all the pain and suffering of the world, and it goes on and on until the person surrenders to the fact that they are stuck and it will never stop. Like an alcoholic in a state of hitting rock bottom, there is a complete surrender, and the suffering is then relieved.

Surrender is the key, as the medicine taught me in Session #5. There seems to be a slight difference between saying it with words and doing it. The final surrender is common to the guidelines that have been established for AA [Alcoholics Anonymous] (and other 12-step programs) where "six of the 12 AA steps are related to a higher power and surrendering to it."

Many of my years were spent with a friend who was an alcoholic and took his life at 48 years old. He would continuously chant the words that he had "hit rock bottom," which means ready to surrender. I would believe the words and get taken for a ride again and again.

Nature

I share the belief of many of my contemporaries that the spiritual crisis pervading all spheres of Western industrial society can be remedied only by a change in our worldview. We shall have to shift from the materialistic, dualistic belief that people and their environment are separate toward a new consciousness of an all-encompassing reality, which embraces the experiencing ego, a reality in which people feel their Oneness with animate nature and all of creation.
-Swiss chemist, Albert Hofmann

One of the prevalent feelings described as an outcome of psilocybin and other psychedelic use is an increased desire to love and protect nature. This has not been my experience, as I have not done it outside. A few people have pointed out the nature connection as being important.

Albert Hofmann, the first person to synthesize, ingest, and learn of the psychedelic effects of lysergic acid diethylamide (LSD), stated:

Through my LSD experience and my new picture of reality, I became aware of the wonder of creation, the magnificence of nature, and the animal and plant kingdom. I became very sensitive to what will happen to all this and all of us.

Journalist Michael Pollan tried psilocybin after talking to dying cancer patients in a Johns Hopkins study of psilocybin and end-of-life anxiety. He took it in his garden and described:

> *I had a fairly high-dose experience in my garden, and I had a very strong sense of the plant—that consciousness was spread more equally over the natural world than I had ever thought before. I was gazing at these leaves; these leaves were gazing back at me, with incredible benign effect. But that everything was much more alive than it had ever been.*[53]

In one study directly related to the nature psilocybin connection, researchers discovered:

> *The psychedelic experience made participants feel more connected to the natural world. These effects continued long after intoxication effects wore off, contributing to a greater sense of wellbeing.*[54]

The nature connection carries over to other psychedelics; in an article on the strong relationship between LSD and nature, author Tessa Love wrote:

> *Psychologists Stanley Krippner and David Luke hypothesized that the consumption of psychedelics creates a greater concern for ecological issues. Several other psychologists have even argued that psychedelic drugs were the catalyst for the environmental movement that sprung up in the late 1960s.*[55]

Stanislav Grof described subjects "undergoing (the 1950s) LSD therapy sessions reporting a dissolution of boundaries and awe-inducing feelings of unity with nature during peak psychedelic effects."

Strangely, this same concern for nature seems to be a part of the experience of many people who declare they have been inside a UFO. Many experiencers report being shown a screen where they are forced to watch images of the earth being destroyed by ecological devastation.

Young children at school in Ruwa, Zimbabwe, also reported the same ecological theme in 1994, where numerous children saw a UFO land. A couple of aliens then walked around the schoolyard. The children reported that they received images in their heads showing the ecological destruction of the Earth.

Death of Materialism

Twenty-five percent were atheists before their DMT experience, but only 7 percent were after.
- 2019 Johns Hopkins Center for Psychedelic & Consciousness Research Paper

What quantum physics teaches us is that everything we thought was physical is not physical.
-Dr. Bruce Lipton

Most people who have taken high-dose psilocybin, high-dose LSD, DMT, or 5-MeO-DMT, will describe that there appears to be some mystical, non-physical component to what they experienced. Research on psilocybin done at Johns Hopkins showed that participants "rated the session as the most spiritually significant experience of their lives, and 80 % rated it among their top five meaningful life experiences."

Many of those who have not had the high-dose psilocybin experience can remain skeptical and relate that the encounters must just be "the brain on drugs."

People treated with high dose psilocybin at places like Johns Hopkins, NYU, or King's College London, come out of the experience with rewired brains. Results include 80% of people who have a six-month abstinence rate from smoking, or 80% with six months sustained decreases in depression and anxiety in patients with life-threatening cancer, or the 80% six months success rate with psilocybin and MDMA against PTSD, or the 70% alcoholic cure rate claimed by some working with LSD, mescaline, or psilocybin.

So how does this relate to materialism? The modern world is now run by science, and most of those scientists adopt the mechanistic, materialistic model. More importantly, an extremely high percentage of scientists believe the random evolutionary model that we are chemical and biological robots in a random, meaningless universe. In this evolutionary mechanistic model, there is no God. The universe is just a pointless process of rolling the dice devoid of spiritual superstitions. Stephen Hawking summed it up, stating, "One can't prove that God doesn't exist. But science makes God unnecessary. ... The laws of physics can explain the universe without the need for a creator."

In a survey conducted by the Pew Research Center for the People & the Press in 2009 of scientists who are members of the American Association for the Advancement of Science, it was found that members, on the whole, were much less religious than the general public.

The number of scientists who identified themselves as atheists was 41% compared to 4% in the American public. The National Academy of Sciences rates, where the big high priests of science reside, the situation is even more acute. Larson and Witham (1998) found that 92% of the National Academy of Sciences members reject a belief in God or higher power.[56] (For people who have trouble with numbers-it is just about all of them.)

Most of these scientists would see themselves as rational and analytical, devoid of being held by the trap of beliefs. They believe that left-brain thinking, based solely on objectively collected evidence, is how they came to disregard a higher power concept. They would say that they simply followed the scientific evidence. Is this belief verifiable or accurate?

Consider the results of the psilocybin tests done at Johns Hopkins University of subjects that did high dose psilocybin for anxiety, depression, or addiction. It was discovered that just like the subjects who no longer smoked, or were depressed, or addicted, the atheists were no longer atheists by almost the same percentage after their brain was rewired. After one high dose session, 57% no longer associated with an atheist belief. Through subjective experience, they suddenly believed there was some sort of entity beyond their believing brain:

> *The most common descriptive labels for the entity were: a being, guide, spirit, alien, and helper. Although 41% of respondents reported fear during the encounter, the most prominent emotions both in the respondent and attributed to the entity were love, kindness, and joy. Most respondents endorsed that the entity had the attributes of being conscious, intelligent, and benevolent, existed in some real but different dimensions of reality and continued to exist after the encounter. Respondents endorsed receiving a message (69%) or a prediction about the future (19%) from the experience. More than half of those who identified as an atheist before the experience no longer identified as atheist afterward. The experiences were rated as among the most meaningful, spiritual, and psychologically insightful lifetime experiences, with persisting positive changes in life satisfaction, purpose, and meaning attributed to the experiences.[57]*

Here are the results of an anonymous online survey of 4,285 people, reporting DMT or non-psychedelic, mystical experiences, conducted by the psychiatry and neuroscience researchers at the Johns Hopkins University School of Medicine and published in PLOS One:

> *One of the paper's most striking findings is that people who identified as atheists dropped that identity after a psychedelic encounter with*

something that felt greater than themselves. Twenty-one percent of the psychedelic users reported being atheists before their experience, while only 8 percent reported being atheists after. The biggest absolute change in atheist status occurred after mystical encounters induced by DMT: 25 percent were atheists before their experience, versus only 7 percent after.[58]

One high dose psilocybin session and their subjective beliefs were gone. As one article described it, they had found "God" or "ultimate reality." The results strongly indicate that atheism is nothing more than a mental health challenge. It can be cured, just like those who used psilocybin to treat alcohol/drug addiction, depression, anxiety, anorexia, and bulimia nervosa.

Skeptical atheists would counter that there was still a percentage who remained atheists. Still, if it was a rational, analytic conclusion that there is no higher power, no one should be jumping ship after a couple of minutes with DMT.

The Guide

I have never met anyone who's had a flashback in my life, and I took millions of trips in the sixties, and I have never met anyone who has had a problem. I have had bad trips, but I have had bad trips in life. I have had a bad trip on a joint. I can get paranoid just sitting in a restaurant; I do not have to take anything.

-John Lennon

One of the protocols that I might be challenged on is not using a guide. Many consider it to be a part of the proper set and setting. Usually, the idea is that this person should be someone who is trusted. In the research setting, a male and female therapist sits with you for the whole 6-hour session. In a legalized psilocybin world, these guides will be part of the protocol, and sessions will not be cheap.[10]

Every one I could find explained why this is necessary. At first glance, it sounds like the ego brings fear and conservatism into the equation. One of the main reasons for my not using a guide is that I have never talked to anyone in my direct group of friends about it.

Jim Fadiman insists that everyone should use a guide. I carefully listened when he explained why a guide should be there. He mentioned things like directing people to the bathroom or advising people not to eat things that are not food. I thought, "Really, that is what they do? I will invite someone to my bedroom to be there if a forget where the bathroom is?"

He also mentioned a situation where a girl was stoned and driving home and suddenly realized that she did not know what a car or a road was. That appeared to me to be more of a problem with the set and setting. My set and setting were my bedroom, lying down with a headset and music. Anything that

---

[10] Other costs will involve the actual facilitator of the session, the cost of the room, an on-call Dr., insurance, and the cost of the pure psilocybin for which there are now only two producers with patent rights.

involved moving from location to location should have been eliminated before these people began to trip.

Another issue everyone brings up is the "bad trip." My second trip looked like it was going to be one of those when it started. The bad trip ended when I took responsibility for what was happening and started talking and describing what was happening as an observer.

The bad trip is one of the reasons that people use to have a guide who can tell you that everything is okay:

> *Psychedelics acts as an opener. However, you open into the situation that you are in, and you are very sensitive to it. When we talk about a set and setting, we mean what is your emotion likelihood or sensitivity, or intention. That turns out to be very critical...what we are finding is that when people have what they call bad trips, which we are replacing with the word challenging, and the reason for that is that people report that they got more total learning about how to be in this world out of the difficult or challenging trip that "good" ones.[59]*

Psychologist Dr. Roland Griffith added to this, saying nothing formed in consciousness can hurt you. It is all consciousness, and we must take responsibility for what we are experiencing rather than blaming demons, psychedelics, or Hillary Clinton.

Victimhood is a significant explanation for the downs we experience in life. It has become commonplace to complain about the dealer attempting to change the cards rather than playing the cards we are dealt with.

A final consideration for using a guide, or not using one, is the level of understanding that the guide has. One example might be a situation where the subject is doing 20 grams. At this level, they will probably go through some dark moments that could look distressing to the guide. If the guide has not experienced 20 grams themselves, there is a good chance they will be phoning 911 when things look like they are out of control when they are not.

A guide is analogous to Reiki healing, or meditation sessions where people are encouraged to visualize surrounding themselves with the white light of protection.

This is the same case that was built for Papal and priestly supremacy in the Roman Catholic church. In 1545, the Catholic Council of Trent declared this: "We define that the Holy Apostolic See and the Roman Pontiff hold primacy over the whole world."

The word of the Pope and priests became inspired by God and could not be questioned. At the same time, they act as mediators or intermediaries to God. They are the shepherds of the sheep. A similar belief structure is built around politicians, who promote themselves as Saviors and Messiahs.

We can use a guide or call in a priest or politician when we have a psilocybin session. We can become like the sheep who are quite vulnerable without a shepherd who will protect them from enemies such as wolves and thieves or protect them from getting lost when they wander from the flock. This may work, but it keeps us victims to the outside evils that may not exist.

The guiding concept sets up the person as a possible victim who may be at risk during the session unless they pay for protection from the guide, politician, healer, or psychic. People are made to believe there are evil forces, evil aliens, and malevolent spirits out there preparing to eat them, probe them, or steal their souls while under the influence unless they pay for protection.

In many ways, the psychedelic guides are playing the fear game, and that fear game is the fastest way to separate someone from their money. For the guide to get the money, the subject must buy into the fear. With no fear, who needs a guide? The conscious left-brain ego has a job to pick up on this manufactured fear and warn its human host that there may be a clear and present danger. The psychedelic guides promote the idea that you could be putting your mind or soul at risk without hiring them.

If a person has researched this topic enough or has orientation on what to expect, they will understand there is no one to blame "out there."

My sense is, "What is an outsider going to do to help me?" They are not in my experience. Everyone I know would not have the foggiest idea about what is happening to me or what to do, except to call 911 when they panic. The concept of a guide, who believes they will rescue you, seems to play into the fear aspect, which is not a good thing to bring along into your trip. Using the guide sets up a belief that something could go wrong, and you will need some help. Anticipating disaster might just manifest disaster. What is feared will appear.

Presenting and then fearing the experience is the worst thing that someone can do, especially if they claim they genuinely know how it works. Nobel Laureate John Wheeler said, "It's a participatory universe," so whatever you bring into the experience has a good chance of manifesting.

"Thoughts are things," said Edgar Cayce and, "the spirit is the life, the mind is the builder, and the physical is the result." We become what we think. There is no separation of me, a good victim here, and the evil forces out there who are waiting to destroy me. We are not victims. We are the captains of our ships and must take ownership.

One concept is that if you have a guide, you can go deeper. This should be seen in context. When the substance is taken, all the emergency exit doors get locked. There is nothing that can be done to stop what is about to happen. The medicine will provide what is needed, and that may be a challenging experience.

A person will not stay on the edge if they do not have a guide. If they are going down a rat hole, they will go there whether they have a guide or not. They go down there in the experience because they are afraid and then resist and fight what is happening rather than surrendering.

The guide can present one essential aid to encourage surrender once a negative scene is experienced. This should be taught before handing the care keys to the client.

A better solution for me is to teach owning the experience, realizing there are no good or bad experiences. They are all just experiences, and we create them. As has been said of bad trips – bad trips are only you learning at a rate you are not accustomed to. Maybe there should be a rule that you get a guide in lesson #1, and then we take the training wheels off the bike. At some point, we must learn to do our homework because, in a way, that is why we are on Earth – to learn.

We need to own whatever happens. Without personal responsibility, there is no growth of character and soul. We need to bring in the understanding that we will learn no matter what happens. When I go in, I take along the expression "nothing inside consciousness can hurt me," and I will be given what is needed. The guide often implies that I will take the good stuff, and someone will rescue me if the experience goes south.

This does not mean that the sessions are a walk in the park. As I have explained before, my ego goes into fear mode before every experience. It tries to talk me out of doing it.

However, as I found with all the 70+ contact modalities, the ego must be quietened and overcome. Otherwise, we will never get into the noetic field where all the information about reality is and where our missions on Earth are stored.

Hallucinatory Reality

All the world's a stage, and all the men and women are but actors. They have their entrances and exits, and each man plays many roles.
-William Shakespeare

LSD does cause psychosis – in the people who do not take it.
-Timothy Leary

The universe does not exist "out there," independent of us. We are inescapably involved in bringing about that which appears to be happening. We are not only observers. We are participators. In some strange sense, this is a participatory universe.
-Physics Nobel Laureate John Wheeler

All the world is a stage, and my experience is that outside of being in the psilocybin state, it is almost impossible to break away from the belief that we are the actor on the stage instead of the observer watching the play. As the mystics say, we forget who we indeed are – and remember who "we" are is what we work to achieve. Instead of reality, we live and breathe in a hallucinatory world created by our five senses.

The term hallucinatory reality is often used by Dennis McKenna. It implies that the experience we have always thought of as the real reality is a hallucination. Our brains are interpreting noisy and ambiguous signals. We are hallucinating all the time, and when we agree on our hallucinations, we call that reality.

Anil Seth is a neuroscience professor and explains in his TED Talk, "Your brain hallucinates consciousness. Right now, billions of neurons in your brain are working together to generate a conscious experience—and not just any conscious experience, your experience of the world around you and of yourself within it."[60]

This idea that there may not be any external world is gaining support, especially considering the discovery of quantum physics ideas that there may not be any such thing as space and time.

Here are a few more thoughts on hallucinatory reality. I raise this discussion because people who have not experienced high dose psilocybin will talk about the brain creating hallucinations, which accounts for what is seen during these altered states.

This notion is negated because I and others will report that the experiences are more real than the 3D world, which seems to be the hallucination if there is one.

Secondly, fMRI scans show that the brain's default mode network is quietened down, and alpha (connected to the state of relaxation) waves are reduced. When that shutdown occurs, the hallucinations we perceive as reality are replaced by other perceptions of reality. The brain modules that created the hallucinatory reality are shut off, and so is the physical self-hallucination we believe to be so real.

The third negation is the fact that "hallucination" is a placeholder. It follows the debunking principle to give it a name and make it go away. Who or what is a hallucination? It is anything that someone chooses not to believe.

Fourthly, the hallucination hypothesis is wanting as there are everyday events taking place in, for example, DMT experiences, where 50% of folks report small conscious beings that interact with the person having the experience.

So how do we know what is real?

People will bring up consensus reality. Consensus reality is that which is generally agreed to be a reality, based on a consensus view. If that is the rule, what was the consensus reality in 1491? It would have been almost a 100% vote for a flat earth at the center of the Universe, with the sun revolving around the Earth. The only things that would exist if we believed this hypothesis are things we see which are solid and measurable.

In the psychedelic world, almost everyone doing high dose psilocybin will experience the nine states of a mystical experience, and none of these exist in the conscious 3D world. Most people doing DMT will encounter small elf-like creatures who come up to meet and greet you. These do not exist in the conscious 3D world, and when they were first reported in the 1990 experiments done by Dr. Strassman, he kept the existence of the beings in the trip reports out of the public literature.

How about the idea that the reality must be predictable, reproducible in an experiment, and measurable? In 1491, putting a level anywhere on the Earth would show the bubble in the middle of the level, indicating the world is flat. The experiment would be reproducible. You could go anywhere on the flat Earth and get the same result.

In the same way, the belief about the Sun revolving around the Earth was highly predictable and measurable. The alignment of the Stonehenge and the Pyramids indicates that the ability to predict when and where the Sun would rise and set was well documented even by the earliest civilizations.

Do the measurement and predictability mean the world is flat with the sun revoting around the Earth every day?

The fact is that our view of reality has continuously changed over the centuries. The big question is, "Has the world become more woo-woo, or more materialistic as we have learned new things?" There could be many examples given, but here are a few that strongly indicate that the world has become less nuts and bolts like and more like the Maya concept described by ancient Hindu scriptures as:

> *The world is an illusion, a play of the supreme consciousness of God. It is a projection of things and forms that are temporarily phenomenal and sustains the illusion of Oneness and permanence. The illusion of the phenomenal world is created and sustained by standalone objects thrown together either by an act of randomness or through the deliberate choice of conscious will.*[61]

- Science once perceived only five thousand stars and executed Giordano Bruno, the Italian philosopher, in 1600. He was burned alive in Rome by those rational, analytical scientists as a heretic for saying the universe has no center, and stars are suns, surrounded by planets and moons.
- The idea of a flat earth at the center of the Universe with a few stars around it has been replaced with an endless universe. In the mystical state experienced

with psilocybin, this is experienced as an ecstatic feeling created by "an overwhelming sense of awe at "your" (now non-existent) insignificance in comparison to the vastness of existence."

- Science once believed that atoms were solid and indivisible. That all ended in 1899. Ernest Rutherford ran the now-infamous gold foil experiment where he determined that the atom was not a solid elementary building block of the universe and made almost entirely of space. There is still a strong following of believers who think that matter is solid. It is one of the critical reasons for a skeptic to doubt the UFO experiencer story of being taken through their home's walls and into a UFO.

- A few years after this discovery, Neils Bohr won the Nobel Prize that recognized his work on atoms' structure. He took the basic building block of the materialistic paradigm and went straight to woo-woo. He said, "Everything we call real is made of things that cannot be regarded as real." That may be why he was a great follower of the Hindu Vedas and said, "I go into the Upanishads to ask questions."[62]

- Not surprisingly, Hinduism has a history of psychedelic use going back to the Vedic time. The oldest scriptures of Hinduism, the Rig Veda, mentions ritualistic consumption of a divine psychedelic known as Soma. The wisdom of the Soma educated the Hindus on actual reality. They, in turn, influenced the thoughts of crucial quantum physics pioneers such as Werner Heisenberg, Niels Bohr, and Erwin Schrödinger. Schrödinger, who won the Nobel prize for coming up with his famous wave equation that predicts how the quantum mechanical wave function changes with time, stated, "After the conversations about Indian philosophy, some of the ideas of Quantum Physics that had seemed so crazy suddenly made much more sense."

- The quantum physics world also introduces the connection to consciousness and the total castration of the materialistic worldview. At this point, the concepts of Oneness, eternal self, and the idea that consciousness is primary are all used interchangeably by the quantum mechanics pioneers, Hinduism, Buddhism, and those who have traveled into the psychedelic non-dual states. Here are some of the more various quotes from the leading quantum mechanics pioneers.

   Schrödinger - 'There is no kind of framework within which we can find consciousness in the plural; this is simply something we construct because of the temporal plurality of individuals, but it is a false construction. The only solution to this conflict insofar as any is available to us at all lies in the ancient wisdom of the Upanishad.'

   Werner Heisenberg, the physicist, who came up with the uncertainty principle, stated, "Of course, we all know that our reality depends on the structure of our consciousness; we can objectify no more than a small part of our world."

Max Planck, Nobel Laureate and the originator of Quantum theory - "I regard consciousness as fundamental. I regard matter as derivative from consciousness. We cannot get behind consciousness. Everything that we talk about, everything that we regard as existing, postulates consciousness."

Niels Bohr physicist - "It still makes no difference whether the observer is a man, an animal, or a piece of apparatus, but it is no longer possible to make predictions without reference to the observer or the means of observation."

John Wheeler, Nobel Laureate who created the concept of wormholes and the term 'black holes' - "No phenomenon is a physical phenomenon until it is an observed phenomenon," and "we are participants in bringing into being not only the near and here, but the far away and long ago," and "We are not only observers. We are participators. In some strange sense, this is a participatory universe."

Eugene Wigner, Nobel Laureate - "When the province of physical theory was extended to encompass microscopic phenomena through the creation of quantum mechanics, the concept of consciousness came to the fore again. It was not possible to formulate the laws of quantum mechanics in a fully consistent way without reference to the consciousness," and "It will remain remarkable, in whatever way our future concepts may develop, that the very study of the external world led to the scientific conclusion that the content of the consciousness is the ultimate universal reality."

- Recent neuroscience has pointed out scores of things that indicate reality is not what it seems. For example, a movie that is a series of still frames being moved at high speed makes it appear to be in motion. This was known already in the late nineteen hundreds. Neurologists have other experiments where they show checkerboards where it seems two squares are the same color when they are not or two lines that appear to be different lengths when they are the same length.

- Next, we have discovered x-rays, electricity, radio waves, TV waves, and the fact we only see a tiny portion of the electromagnetic spectrum. This introduced the invisible realm talked about by mystics for centuries. It also brings in Nikola Tesla, who ditches the material world, saying, "If you wish to understand the universe, think of energy, frequency, and vibration!" These have been vital words of mystics for centuries as well. They are words often used often in psychedelic trip reports.

- Thomas Young's 1804 dual slit experiment showed the principle of particle duality. When Young shone light through two slits, he saw the wave pattern on the back wall indicating a wave pattern directly opposed to Isaac Newton's idea that light was made of particles. The real implications of consciousness's influence did not start until 1961 when Claus Jönsson from the University of Tübingen in Germany machined a set of slits 300 nm wide into copper and then irradiated them with a 40 keV beam of electrons from an electron microscope. In 2013, the experiment was done with single electrons still showing the wave-particle duality.

This led to the notion that the quantum wavefunction is "collapsed" by what he called a psychophysical interaction. In other words, when the experiment is not watched, a wave pattern will appear on the back wall behind the two slits, but when the experiment was observed, it would turn into a particle. The particle remained in a wave in a quantum state if not observed or measured.[11]

Von Neuman was backed up by fellow Eugene Wigner, who stated, "It follows that the quantum description of objects is influenced by impressions entering my consciousness. Solipsism may be logically

---

[11] Time also has nothing to do with it. As Neils Bohr confidently predicted, it makes no difference whether we delay the measurement or not. If we measure the photon's path prior its arrival at a detector is finally registered, we lose all interference. The implication is that nature "knows" not just if we are looking, but if we are planning to look.

consistent with present quantum mechanics." His work was confirmed by John Wheeler, who wrote, "The universe does not exist 'out there,' independent of us. We are inescapably involved in bringing about that which appears to be happening. We are not only observers. We are participators. In some strange sense, this is a participatory universe."

This interpretation, which makes consciousness a crucial part of seeing anything in the physical world, led Einstein to disagree with the observer effect interpretation saying, "I would like to believe the moon is still behind me when I am not looking."[12]

The observer effect's essential connection to psychedelics is that *psychedelic* means mind-manifesting, which exactly is what the observer effect implies. Nothing exists until the observer manifests it into existence from the universal quantum field. This would apply to the physical, dream, NDE, and psychedelic worlds.

Even I experienced this in my sessions. When you focus on something, it comes into being. The process is much more evident under the influence, probably because everyone knows events in the psychedelic state are much more plastic.

The effect was most noticeable to me when taking off my blindfold and headphones to go to the bathroom. I could feel and see the physical world coming back online, and it was a very jarring experience.

This psyche-manifested-reality-concept is why guides are told not to talk but to suggest things to you while sitting with someone in a session (i.e., "You are fine"). With merely a suggestion, it can direct the mind to manifest what they are talking about.

Some will suggest that manifesting under the influence is different from the manifesting of matter out of the quantum field in the 3D world. This, however, is nonsensical. It is all the same consciousness creating both realities. It is ALL MIND MANIFESTED, and it is a typical report by people under the influence of psychedelics that what they view in the psychedelic state is more real than the 3D consciousness.

- 1956 – Peter Safar and James Elam invented mouth-to-mouth resuscitation. The next year a team at Johns Hopkins unveiled the first portable external defibrillator. History will record this as one of the most significant discoveries to help break down the hallucinatory reality that the world had bought into. The techniques and equipment enabled doctors and first responders to bring back people with flatline EEG, which indicates that the brain is no longer involved in creating and interpreting reality.

By 1975, the first book about NDEs, *Life After Life,* was published. Psychiatrist Dr. Raymond Moody wrote it. It was a report on 150 people who were interviewed in a qualitative study of people who had undergone near-death experiences (NDEs). The latest figure is that 15 million Americans have had a near-death experience, there are thousands of books, and the term has become a household word.

What happened is that people started to report near-death experiences indicating that although the brain was entirely offline, the mind was still alive and well. Those documented realities were much more real and vivid than subjective, waking, hallucinatory reality. More importantly, the still-active mind was reporting a world that was very much like the psychedelic world. Reports came back stating that everything is One, feelings of unconditional love, an encounter with non-earthly beings, and themes related to death and dying.

One study on the connection between NDEs and the psychedelic drug DMT concluded, "Results revealed significant increases in phenomenological features associated with the NDE, following DMT administration compared to placebo. Also, we found significant relationships between the NDE scores and DMT-induced, ego-dissolution and mystical-type experiences and a significant association between NDE scores and baseline trait 'absorption' and delusional ideation measured at baseline. Furthermore, we found a significant overlap in nearly all the NDE phenomenological features when comparing DMT-induced NDEs with a matched group of 'actual' NDE experiencers. These results reveal a striking similarity between these states that warrants further investigation."[63]

The correlation is significant as it strongly indicates that new, higher reality states can be caused by shutting down the brain or deactivating the brain, as was recorded in the research done at Imperial College London. Like the shutting down of the brain during an NDE,[13] the London researchers reported on patients taking psilocybin "decreased activity and connectivity in the brain's key connector hubs, enabling a state of unconstrained cognition."[64]

Furthermore, it confirms the evidence that the brain itself is causing hallucinatory reality. When it is taken offline with an NDE or psychedelic, the "still active mind" can view an unfiltered reality that may be closer to the truth.

- Holographic Universe - The holographic universe idea that came in conjunction with the concept was that the holographic brain. The idea that arose was that the universe is a hologram, and the brain is a hologram tuner.

---

[13] Material mind=brain. Neurologists will try and argue that the brain is not offline despite the flatline, but the psilocybin research indicates it does not have to be completely shut down, just quietened down or moved out of the way.

The Psychedelic Multi-Vitamin

Modern science has become fascinated by the materialistic paradigm. This means that the human is seen as a chemical, biological robot in a random, meaningless universe.

The medical and drug industries have adopted this paradigm. That is why when someone gets sick, they are given a chemical to handle their health problem. The body is seen as a chemical factory that has gone wrong, so chemicals are the apparent choice for correcting the situation.

This ideology has made its way into the world of psychedelics. All the scientifically accepted research done on psychedelics today is conducted by pharmacologists who are in the business of making pharmacy drugs to market to the public.

That is why synthetic psilocybin is now being used instead of the natural mushroom. Instead of eating vegetables and fruit, the pharmaceutical solution is to produce a multivitamin with all of the 'active' ingredients.

Researchers will say that the synthetic chemical will be purer than the street mushrooms. Secondly, they will argue that you must have a refined product that can be accurately measured to do good science, so everyone gets the same dose. Those who are in favor of legalizing psilocybin are so vested in their pursuit that they look the other way when it comes to what is used in laboratory trials. The doctors and pharmaceutical companies will encourage the move to chemicals as they will control what is made, how it is made, what it is used for, and receive all the money earned from its sales.

Psychedelic mushrooms contain beta-carboline MOAI alkaloids, baeocystin, phenylethylamine, serotonin, aeruginascin, and other compounds that have not been studied, due to the illegal status of the mushrooms. Researchers have chosen to ignore everything except psilocybin, which would be marketed, and the profits will be added to the pharmaceutical companies' trillions. If and when psilocybin becomes public, it will be sold as the chemical "equivalent" and not a magic mushroom.

Many in the psychedelic field talk about the mushrooms' wisdom and how it has been unearthed as fossilized fungi dating back to up to one billion years. Many also believe that the mushroom's wisdom is passed down, which would mean that taking mushrooms would allow a billion years of knowledge to be shared. In the same vein, pure synthetic psilocybin may have only days or months of wisdom, if any.

A second consideration is that mushrooms may carry a frequency with their strain. Most psychedelics have similar chemical structures, but they allow for separate lessons and a different learning atmosphere. A mushroom trip is much different than an LSD trip, which is much different from a 5-MeO-DMT trip, which is very different from DMT, and so on.

If this is all true, it will all be reduced to a psilocybin trip with limited benefits.

The Professional Question

> *"Now, do you see? Now, do you see?"*
> **-Dr. Rick Strassman describes the message he got from the DMT beings.**

> *Now one of the things that you have noticed is that there's no science yet—just worldwide use.*
> **-Dr. Jim Fadiman on micro-dosing psychedelics.**

> *What people sometimes don't get about science is that we often have phenomena that remain unexplained.*
> **-MIT astrophysicist Sara Seager**

One of my research friends in the UFO community asked a former high-level intelligence official, "What could I say that would make you so angry that you would no longer talk to me?" He replied, "Mess with the money." People must keep in mind that money is the primary and overriding rule, especially in a capitalist system.

Many professional researchers dealing with psychedelics will claim that they can be dangerous. Fear of danger has helped create a situation where the authorities have criminalized nature and where you <u>can</u> be arrested if the wrong mushroom species pops up on your front lawn. The War on Drugs propaganda was put out by President Richard

Nixon, which he used to target his enemies who were opposed to his war in Vietnam.

Additionally, we are told that psychedelics should only be taken and researched under the strict protocols of a lab where there is extensive pre-screening, preparatory training, two therapists in the room, a Dr. on standby, and synthesized psilocybin instead of the natural mushroom. Many experts speak against people doing it without the proper set and setting, as there are many risks.

The modern psychedelic worldview also points out that psychedelic use is illegal and that only those who have a license to administer the psychedelic can distribute it. That may make the subject feel better, but it is costly. Moreover, people who might want to explore the benefits cannot get into a study because there is not much research being done. Therefore, the number of subjects taken is exceptionally low.

This advice to the public is remarkably like religious practices of the past where the priestly class made rules that the common class should be told what is true. Now, the modern, scientific, priestly class is doing the same thing. Some examples:

- In the Old Testament's Book of Exodus, Moses ordained public readings of the Torah by the day's high priests. Jewish Roman historian Flavius Josephus described the rules: "...every week men should desert their other occupations and assemble to listen to the Torah and to obtain a thorough and accurate knowledge."

- Most people are aware that the New Testament books consist only of those 27 books sanctioned by the Synod of Hippo 393 C.E. and four years later by the Council of Cartage. Some books were considered inspired by God, and the rest were banned.
- The early Christian Church discouraged the populace from reading the Bible on their own. That policy deepened through the Middle Ages and later. There was even a prohibition forbidding the translation of the Bible into native languages.

Religious high priests of the past and professional researchers must be like politicians. As politicians, they are reactive to the weather of the day. It has to be that way because they convince foundations or drug companies to put up the enormous amounts of money required to do the rigorous double-blind studies and produce the papers for journals.

The question that needs to be asked is, "Who is producing the weather?" It is not professional researchers. It is the people on the street. They produce the weather.

There is a famous story that Bill Wilson, one of the founders of AA, encouraged LSD research in the 1950s. He had been told stories from alcoholics that they never touched a drink after taking LSD. He was determined to help those alcoholics who could not "get the spiritual," which is a crucial component of the AA Twelve Steps. No official study was ever done.

Bill Wilson was not the only one promoting LSD for alcohol recovery. Aldous Huxley, doing LSD research at Harvard, wrote to Father Thomas Merton, who ran a Trappist Monastery in Kentucky. The Abby hosted a yearly AA gathering, and Merton was one of the top Roman Catholic writers of the time on spirituality and social justice. Huxley to Merton in 1959 wrote about his friend Bill Wilson:

> *A friend of mine, saved from alcoholism during the last fatal phases of the disease, by a spontaneous theophany which changed his life as completely as St. Paul's was changed on the road to Damascus, has taken lysergic acid two or three times and affirms that his experience under the drug is identical with the spontaneous experience which changed his life – the only difference being that the spontaneous experience did not last so long as the chemically induced one. There is, obviously, a field here for serious and reverent experimentation.*[65]

Seventy years later, some Universities like NYU are doing high-dose psilocybin studies to test the theory that alcoholism can be eliminated in many people suffering from the condition. They are using a dose of 40mg/70kg. These studies were already conducted 70 years ago with LSD. Saskatchewan researchers Doctors Abram Hoffer and Humphrey Osmond began investigations in 1952 with alcoholism and LSD and reported one study with a recovery rate of 70%.[66]

Where did the researchers get the idea to do the present drinking/LSD study? They did not think it up. They heard the rumor on the street about people being helped and decided to fund research to confirm or deny the stories and then sell the treatment to the alcoholic community. The researchers are reactive.

In the same way, numerous studies are being done at universities looking at the idea that high-dose psilocybin can treat smoking, cocaine, and heroin addictions. One smoking study was done, and they came up with an 80% abstinence rate after six months compared to Nicotine patches with a ~20% abstinence rate. There would have been no smoking study had it not been for regular people finding out this benefit through experimentation.

The same is true for many of the other studies that have been proposed or are in progress. Psilocybin studies are being initiated regarding treatment-resistant depression, addictions, anorexia nervosa, and existential distress caused by a life-threatening disease. They are just following up on research done on the street.

Another example to illustrate the point is the practice of microdosing with LSD or psilocybin. This is all the rage right now and is creating the weather that will become future studies. Microdosing claims benefits such as, improved mood, increased creativity, decreased trauma, relief of anxiety, decrease the need for caffeine, less procrastination, reduced depression, help with PTSD, PSM, autism, a few reports of help with stuttering, writer's block, workflow, and a host of other claims.

Jim Fadiman, one of the most knowledgeable people in the world on the subject, was asked if there is any controlled research being done on the subject. He stated the answer used to be "No," but there is a little bit now. In another lecture, he jokingly said, "There is no science yet. Just worldwide use."

As articles and claims about the benefits increase, the weather will become more severe. Capitalist companies will see a benefit to using microdosing to make their workers/slaves more efficient. The laboratories will be able to sell study proposals, and other laboratories will check out the claims.

Big-name university labs and drug companies are just followers. They wait for the regular Joe on the street to start a parade. When the numbers create demand, they then race to lead the parade. The role of the regular Joe should never be underestimated or minimized.

That is why the same pharmaceutical companies promoting antidepressants are now busy with their legal teams filing broad patents on all the potential intellectual property surrounding psychedelic synthetic molecules. The compounds are patented and then will be commercialized. These patents will prevent others from entering the field.

The practice is run from a playbook that drug companies have used for decades. The small researchers will not survive in this kind of atmosphere. It will be a land-grab world like the rest of the drug world, where there are only a couple of players.

In doing many sessions, I realized a big difference from my eyes being open to what I regularly experienced, under the covers, with music and a blindfold on. I would not have known the difference unless I had done so many sessions and had to use the bathroom so many times.

The psychedelic state can be controlled to a great extent, and there is a considerable difference in the experience, whether you have your eyes opened or eyes closed. After many times reverting from one state to another, it seemed that I could control, to an extent, the condition that I was in.

Test subjects in university studies only do it once or twice. Therefore, they never learn to control what is happening. The data produced is missing the fact that the positive and negative effects can be directed, to an extent, with experience. They are simply documenting what is happening in naïve users.

University research is 50 years behind what is happening in the public arena, so it will be many years until research shows methods and techniques that will help manage the psilocybin state.

A final problem with psychedelic research by pharmacologists and psychiatrists is that they have a problem experiencing the drugs they claim expertise in.

For example, Rick Strassman is a pharmacologist who did an extensive study on DMT in the 1990s. He had a DMT experience, which led him to begin his research. Strassman wrote about "Jacob," the volunteer, who had an experience where he saw the DMT beings (or machine elves as Terence McKenna called them) emerged from a raging psychedelic waterfall, asking him in a sing-song manner, "Now do you see? Now, do you see?" Could this volunteer be Strassman?

When I first smoked DMT, these little beings, maybe three or four feet tall, merged from a flaming waterfall. There were flaming colors that comprised the waterfall. These little beings that I would describe as aliens if I were to refer to them in any way. They said, 'Now do you see? Now, do you see? Now, do you see?' Just over and over again. As a result of that vision, I was set on course to study DMT and then to follow it wherever it led with the information and the data in a way that individual tip of being asked over and over 'Now do you see?' It changed my life. It infuses my activity in my academic career.[67]

Most of the time, however, Strassman does not answer the question. In one podcast, he said:

Well, that is a question I am asked a lot... It is a question I sidestep by saying if I tell people I have, I am accused of being a zealot, and if I say I haven't, then I am accused of not knowing what I am talking about.[68]

That may be why when Strassman told the story in the epilogue of his book *DMT: The Spirit Molecule,* it was made to appear that it was one of the volunteers, Saul, a 32-year-old married psychologist, for the study that had provided the story:

Out of the raging, colossal waterfall of flaming color expanding into my visual field, the roaring silence and unspeakable joy, they stepped, or rather, emerged. Welcoming, curious, they almost sang, "Now do you see?" I felt their question pour into and fill every possible corner of my awareness: "Now do you see? Now, do you see?" Trilling, sing-song voices, exerting enormous pressure on my mind.

There was no need to answer. It was as if someone had asked me, on a blazing cloudless midsummer afternoon in the New Mexico desert, "Is it bright? Is it bright?" The question and the answer are identical. Added to my "Yes!" was a deeper "Of course!" And finally, an intensely poignant "At last!"[69]

Despite his experience, Strassman usually avoids the question of whether or not he has done DMT. Scientists are afraid that they will be seen either as no longer independent of what they are studying or as drug addicts as they will indeed be judged.

The problem with scientists not taking the psychedelic that is being studied is that they quickly become like the Pope moralizing sex and marriage for the Roman Catholic church. How can you comment on something you know nothing about?

William James talked about this ineffable quality of the mystical state and how it will evade anyone who has not been there:

Mystical states are more like states of feeling than like states of intellect. No one can make clear to another who has never had a certain feeling, in what the quality or worth of it consists. One must have musical ears to know the value of a symphony; one must have been in love with one's self to understand a lover's state of mind.[70]

Interdisciplinary Solution

N ow science is looking towards clinical pharmacologists to solve the mystery of psychedelics. Although, as pointed out above, the process is prolonged, expensive, and subject to being consumed by those funding the research's ultimate financial interests.

The second main problem of not treating this in an interdisciplinary way is the problem of stovepiping. This is the main reason why science has not solved the UFO problem for 73 years, even though they have probably had hardware from the craft and alien bodies from the crashes for the entire time.

In the reductionist system used by science, the main problem has been that the UFOs and the other evidence have been hampered by security classifications and stovepiping. Each small part of the evidence has been portioned out to various faculties with specialists like physics, engineering, chemistry, and the military.

Because of the subject's classification, none of the specialists are talking to the others. The craft and its occupants, as many experiencers describe, are a single unit that works together.

There are a couple of hundred faculties of study, and neuropharmacology is only one of them. People forget that PhDs in this field cannot necessarily fly a plane, fix a toilet, understand physics, meditation, or cooking. People assume that because they have a PH. D, they are so smart they must know everything. This is extremely far from the truth.[71]

They know a lot about extraordinarily little, but in many cases, they believe their field of study has all the answers for everything. Pharmacologists believe that the secret to understanding psychedelics lies in pharmacology. A priest would think that the answer lies in the Bible, and a police officer might see the answer in the street crime that some drugs cause.

Moreover, the pharmacologist has no time to look at any other field of study for an answer as he is not trained in it. Secondly, if he, as a pharmacologist, were to go down another road looking for the solution, he would lose his job and may end up working at McDonald's. Each field is going to their corner in the issue, as they are the ones paying the bills and believe they have the answer.

As science worships what they call proof, they believe that the evidence has been established, and the conclusion they have arrived at needs no future discussion. Scientists end up in a situation where they know, and others just believe. The fact is that their belief may be closer to reality, but they, too, just believe.

Conclusion

Strassman's important (DMT) research contributes to a growing awareness that we inhabit a multidimensional universe that is far more complex and interesting than the one our scientific theories have shown us. It is of the utmost importance that we face the implications of this discovery, for it has so much to tell us about who we are and why we are here.

-John Mack, former professor and the head of the department of psychiatry at Harvard Medical School

The Sage sees the world as an expansion of his own self. So, what need has he to accumulate things? By giving to others, he gains more and more by serving others; he receives everything Heaven gives, and all things turn out for the best. The Sage lives, and all things go as Tao goes; all things move as the wind blows.

-Final words of the Tao Te Ching

The modern world has developed many techniques to solve problems and explain the reality in which we find ourselves. There are hundreds of different fields that study this, such as physical chemistry, organic chemistry, inorganic chemistry, analytical chemistry, biochemistry, astrophysics, quantum mechanics, atomic physics, molecular physics, nuclear physics, Mechanical engineering, chemical engineering, civil engineering, electrical engineering, electrical management, geotechnical engineering, behavioral psychology, clinical psychology, neuropsychology, child psychology, experimental psychology, and forensic psychology.

Specialties have formed a world of hundreds of little hamster wheels where specialists race along on their own wheel. Their limited worldview forces them to see a problem in a very restricted and narrow way.

Take the example of someone who is depressed. A psychologist would see the solution as talk therapy; a chemist sees everything as chemical-based and would advise a chemical pill to correct a chemical imbalance. Transpersonal psychology would say the answer lies in perhaps holotropic breathwork or psychedelic dose treatment.

Solutions to better understand consciousness and reality must be interdisciplinary. To avoid researching the entire spectrum of evidence would cause the researcher to jump back on his own hamster wheel, going nowhere.

Into this soup of intellectual fields of study come the critical component of noetic information. This information is usually described as coming from outside the rational, analytic mind, which means more from insights, dreams, daydreams, and psychedelic states. It comes with a sense of knowing and a sense of true reality. William James was the first to try and define the state of knowledge that arises saying they, "are states of insight into depths of truth unplumbed by the discursive intellect. They are illuminations, revelations, full of significance and importance, all inarticulate though they remain; and as a rule, they carry with them a curious sense of authority for after-time."

There have been many approaches to solving the problems faced by the modern world, and I believe that psychedelics may be the ultimate solution. It takes us to the world that shamans taught about thousands of years ago. It matches the wisdom of eastern traditions and seems to come from the same place.

Most people in the modern world believe the answer is technology, but I don't see that. The United States has the best technology and has become one of the most dysfunctional countries globally, on the verge of civil war. More technology would be like giving a small child with difficulties a gun. Technology plays well into the belief in separation, which is the underlying problem. In a capitalist society where survival of the fittest is the bottom line, technology only allows the haves to have more control over the have-nots.

Many in the general public will still fear psychedelics and place them in the "drug" category based on the DEA drug schedule that puts them in Schedule 1. Schedule 1 drugs are classified as drugs with no currently accepted medical use and a high potential for abuse.

They do not consider that the FDA calls psychedelic psilocybin a "Breakthrough Therapy" for severe depression and anxiety with an 80% success rate. Nor does the public know that psilocybin is 80% effective in smoking cessation as compared to 17% for present-day therapies.

Psilocybin has also been used with great success for end-of-life anxiety, addiction, treatment-resistant depression, PTSD, and cluster headaches.

Unaware skeptics will point to psychedelics' illegality and will not acknowledge the discoveries made around the latest research in labs worldwide.

The legal argument is only a stop-gap measure. Many areas such as Denver, Oregon, and sections of California have moved to make psilocybin legal or legal for certain psychological conditions. As research shows more and more benefits, clarifies a safe dosage, and there are no addiction factors, it is only a matter of time until the dam breaks, and like the fight against gay marriage, the resistance collapses.

Canada has made great strides in this area. Cannabis is now legal, and it is being used to treat all sorts of conditions. No one jumped off a bridge when it was legalized, and society didn't collapse. Like gambling and liquor, the government collects tax dollars, and that makes it legal and acceptable. Psilocybin is not far behind.

Canadians have made great strides in promoting safe drugs and discouraging the drugs that cause damage to society. The number one killer is cigarettes, which people use to get their nicotine fix. The latest figures show that only

10.8% of Canadians are daily smokers, mainly because it costs over $20.00 per pack.

Likewise, liquor, which is a factor in 40% of all violent crimes today, along with 7% of all traffic accidents, is costly. Combined with massive penalties for impaired driving, this has cut down on the number of people abusing the drug. A simple chart can show the difference between them:

Drug	Condition	Deaths/Year (USA)	Psilocybin & LSD Deaths
Anti-depressants	Depression	48,344 suicides	0 with an 80% success
Nicotine	Lung heart disease	400,000 deaths	Smoking Treatment 0 with an 80% success
Liquor	Accident & violence	95,000 +	LSD 50-90% success

The attitude is quickly changing about psychedelics. Most scientists can do controlled studies on all the disorders that psychedelics claim to cure. Along with those studies are the reports of the spiritual and mystical experiences that go along with stress and depression reduction, smoking cessation, and a PTSD cure.

Lastly, with their incredible access to the internet and the information that can be accessed instantaneously, the new generation is not buying their parents' fear and resistance. They will bring the change as Max Planck, the father of quantum physics, had already discovered over 100 years ago:

> *A new scientific truth does not triumph by convincing its opponents and making them see the light, but rather because its opponents eventually die, and a new generation grows up that is familiar with it.*

A whole new world of medical cures and spiritual discoveries awaits.

Appendix I

The mystical experience is doubly valuable. It is valuable because it gives the experiencer a better understanding of himself and the world and because it may help him live a less self-centered and more creative life.
-Aldous Huxley

The Mystical Experience Questionnaire (MEQ)

This is what researchers use to evaluate whether a participant has had a mystical experience, defined as "the experience of profound unity with all that exists, a felt sense of sacredness, a sense of the experience of truth and reality at a fundamental level (noetic quality), deeply felt positive mood, a transcendence of time and space, and difficulty explaining the experience in words."

The MEQ has been used for more than 50 years. Today's generally accepted version is a 30-item checklist divided into the four categories I've detailed below. The highlights are mine.

Factor 1: Mystical

Freedom from the limitations of yourself and a feeling of unity or a bond with what seems to be something greater than your personal self.

Experience of pure being and pure awareness (beyond the world of sense impressions).

Experience of Oneness concerning an "inner world" within.

Experience the fusion of yourself into a larger whole.

Experience of unity with the ultimate reality.

Feeling that you experienced eternity or infinity.

Experience of Oneness or unity with objects and/or the people perceived in your surroundings.

Experience of the insight that "all is One."

Awareness of a life or living presence in all things.

The gain of insightful knowledge experienced at an intuitive level.

The certainty of encounter with the ultimate reality (in the sense of being able to "know" and "see" what is real at some point during your experience.

You are convinced now, as you look back on your experience, that in it, you encountered ultimate reality (i.e., that you "knew" and "saw" what was really real).

Sense of being at a spiritual height.

Sense of reverence.

Feeling that you experienced something profoundly sacred and holy.

Factor 2: Positive Mood

Experience of amazement.

Feelings of tenderness and gentleness.

Feelings of peace and tranquility.

Experience of ecstasy.

Sense of awe or awesomeness.

Feelings of joy.

Factor 3: Transcendence of Time and Space

Loss of your usual sense of time.

Loss of your usual sense of space.

Loss of usual awareness of where you were.

Sense of being "outside of" time, beyond past and future.

Being in a realm with no space boundaries.

Experience of timelessness.

Factor 4: Ineffability

A sense that the experience cannot be described adequately in words.

Feeling that you could not do justice to your experience by describing it in words.

Feeling it would be challenging to communicate your own experience to others who have not had similar experiences.

Appendix 2

This is a list of states of consciousness used to rate the levels of intensity as reported in psychedelic experiences.

Microdosing (Pre-level 1)

This small dose isn't enough to "trip" in the traditional sense but can lead to subtle yet profound internal shifts. Improvements in mood, productivity, creativity, enhanced focus, less reactivity; and the possibility of relief from depression, anxiety, cluster headaches, and various other symptoms.

Level 1

This level produces a mild "stoned" effect, with some visual enhancement (i.e., brighter colors, etc.) Some short-term memory anomalies. Left/right brain communication changes causing music to sound "wider."

Level 2

With bright colors and visuals (i.e., things start to move and breathe), some 2-dimensional patterns become apparent upon shutting eyes—confused or reminiscent thoughts. Change of short-term memory leads to continual distractive thought patterns. A vast increase in creativity becomes apparent as the natural brain filter is bypassed.

Level 3

Obvious visuals; everything looks curved and/or warped, patterns and kaleidoscopes are seen on walls, with possible faces, etc. Some mild hallucinations such as rivers flowing in wood grain or "mother of pearl" surfaces. Closed eye hallucinations become three-dimensional. There is some confusion of the senses (i.e., seeing sounds as colors, etc.). Time distortions and "moments of eternity."

Level 4

Intense hallucinations (i.e., objects morph into other objects.) Destruction or multiple splitting of the ego. (Things start talking to you, or you find that you are feeling contradictory things simultaneously). Some loss of reality. Time becomes meaningless, out-of-body experiences and E.S.P.-type phenomena. There is a blending of the senses.

Level 5

Total loss of visual connection with reality. The senses cease to function in the usual way. Complete loss of ego. A merging with space, other objects, or the universe. The loss of reality becomes so severe that it defies explanation. The earlier levels are relatively easy to explain in terms of measurable changes in perception and thought patterns. This level is different because the actual universe within which things are typically perceived ceases to exist! Satori enlightenment (and other such labels). [72]

Appendix 3

My Protocols

These are my protocols for the record. Others may have different methods that might work better.

1) **Intention** – People have all sorts of purposes going in. I intended to see the entire process as going to school to learn something. The medicine will give you what you need, not what you want. The whole trip may be conducted by one's higher self instead of some separate, outside force influencing the situation. There is only one thing, and as John Wheeler stated, there is "no out there." We are not corks floating down the stream being buffeted by the waves around us. In this theory, the psilocybin simply shuts down the brain circuits, causing a higher self-blockage. Another way of looking at it is that the psilocybin sends Mr. Stupid (your left brain) for coffee while the lesson is taking place.

2) **In your bedroom or at least lying down** - Some people talk about driving or running around outside. Anyone who is doing anything but lying

down and going within will reap whatever ill that befalls them.

3) **Stay still** - This is something I try to follow as closely as possible. Any movement gives the conscious mind a reason to get involved. It thinks you are awake when your hands and legs are moving. That makes the left brain more active in showing up and beginning to run things. The same principle is used in trying to achieve an out-of-body experience or in remembering a dream. The idea is to get the mind awake and the body asleep.

4) **Own it** – This is the most important thing I try to remember. It's just an experience in consciousness, and I chose to go there. Nothing is more damaging than going into the trip and then spending the entire time playing the victim. Neuroanatomist Jill Bolte Taylor summed it up by saying, "take responsibility for the energy you bring."

5) **Trust, let go, and be open** - This is the mantra given to people in the various Johns Hopkins sessions. I fully believe that any attempt to control the trip is your ego (left brain) trying to stay in control. This is where the dark experiences originate, and it is speculated that this same combative experience leads to negative near-death experiences.

The mind is the creator, and the key is to surrender. Bringing fear into the experience can only lead to trouble. This is expressed in the computer analogy – garbage in, garbage out.

I have yet to have a bad experience, and when the one experience got dark by reminding myself to own the experience, the fear went away. I remind myself that whatever occurs, it will only last five or six hours. I remember that some people live entire lives that are a complete hell, and some of them face imminent death. This puts things in perspective, and the whining child within calms down.

6) **Set a time** – I always set up an exact time when I will start the trip. I use 8:00pm or 3:00am. This reminds me that it is school time and prevents the ego from encouraging us to do it some other time so it can remain in control.

7) **Use a blindfold** – the idea for me is to go within, not observe weird visions while still looking at the physical world. The blindfold also mimics the shamanic ceremonies, which are always done at night in the dark.

Taking the blindfold off to go to the bathroom was a harrowing experience, as seeing the light and the physical world is almost like being thrown into a pool of cold water. Once the blindfold was off, seeing the physical world caused me to be drawn out of the matrix world where my experience had been happening. Needing to use the bathroom is the only instance that would ever get me to take off the blindfold.

8) **Use headphones** – This was especially important. Part of my experience was that I became one with the music and that music drove the experience. When the music was external, such as playing through a speaker in the room, it was harder to become one with it.

9) **Use music** – I use the *Johns Hopkins Psilocybin Playlist* rather than trying to reinvent the wheel. They spent decades setting up the songs that lead you throughout your experience. There is music that fits the intense moments of the experience and music that brings one out of the experience. The music that Johns Hopkins (and other playlists such as NYU) use is instrumental music, rather than songs with English lyrics, perhaps because the language will activate the left brain where the language center is.

10) **Dosage** – There are all sorts of ideas on what kind of dosage to do. To determine your set dose would depend on what you are trying to achieve during the experience. People talk about a *safe dosage*, which means extraordinarily little to me. A vast majority of scientists who do not follow psilocybin research consider psilocybin a DEA Schedule 1 controlled drug and say zero is the only safe dosage. As I was looking for a breakthrough, I preferred the high

dosages of 5 grams and above. The experience is a chance to learn and not a party. My understanding is that the higher the dose, the more intense the experience.

People who have done super high dosages report even deeper trips into the field, where they start to see entities, spirits, and God. Kara, who was doing up to thirteen hits of LSD, reported, "I have never run into anything evil with a capital E. The difficult thing that I have run into is stuff out of my stack. That is the best way that I can put it. I am not saying that cannot exist by that is not something that I have run into...now I have run into saints, spirit guides, golden presences, and sources of light. Those are all great, and I have run into those a lot."

Kilindi Lyi, a Psychonaut who was doing 20-30 grams of mushrooms, reported that the lower 3-gram party doses were "several thousand orders of magnitude away from 20 grams. It's different from the veil that has been pushed aside. Stuff is floating through the room. You are floating through the room on faraway planets and jungles. There are encounters with not just machine elves but also in the insectoids."73

This high dose entity-relationship fits in because entities are reported during trips on morning glory seeds, ayahuasca, and DMT, which are considered high dose encounters.

11) **Tolerance** - is the body's adaptation to the continual presence of a drug. This rule applies not only to psychedelics but substances like alcohol, nicotine, and many others. When we become tolerant, the body requires higher doses to get the previously achieved desired effect. Although there is a tolerance level to psilocybin, the literature on how long to wait between sessions is all over the map. Jim Fadiman, who is an expert on microdosing, advises taking a dose, followed by two days off and another amount on the following day. Johns Hopkins required several weeks between each high dose session when they studied smoking cessation and end-of-life anxiety. I use one week between regular dosage sessions and have had no problem.

12) **Record the session** - I now record all of my sessions as my memory of what happens fades like a dream when the session is over. Recording puts me in an observer status with much less fear. I am merely watching what I am being shown and then describing it. (This same technique is used in hypnosis when the person is reliving a very traumatic or painful experience. The person is told they are just observing, which reduces the trauma and fear.)

13) **Alone or with a guide** – This is a controversial area where people must make their own decision. I

do not use a guide, and that is counter to what most people recommend. I have listened to many protocol recommendations and have not heard any strong reason for using one that makes sense to me. A guide would be necessary to those who have no background or who have not researched this in-depth. Some may find it challenging to have a horde of new things (that do not fit into the usual conscious hallucination) happening one after another.

OTHER BOOKS ON ITSALLCONNECTED PUBLISHING

All available on Amazon as both paperback and eBooks

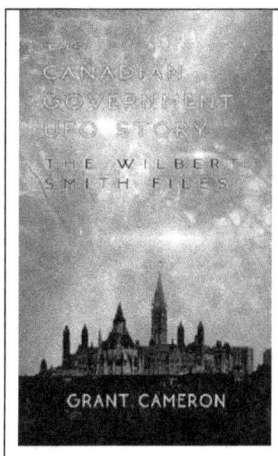	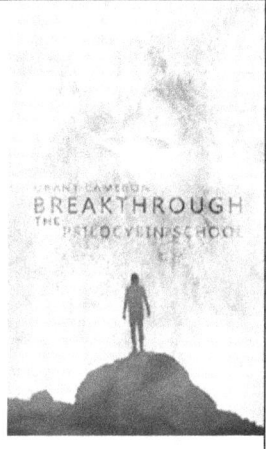	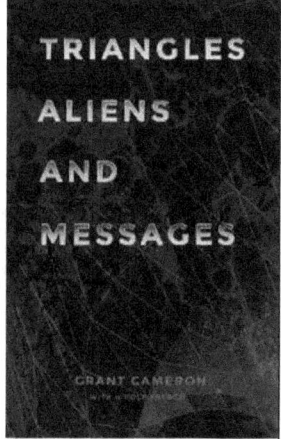
The Canadian UFO Story: Wilbert Smith	Breakthrough: The Psilocybin School	Triangles, Aliens and Messages

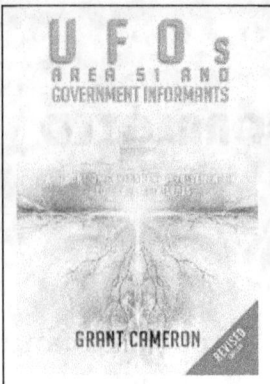	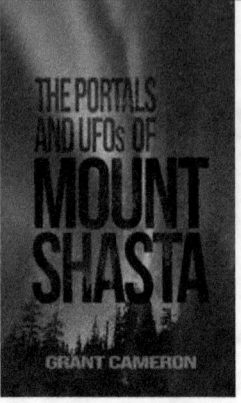	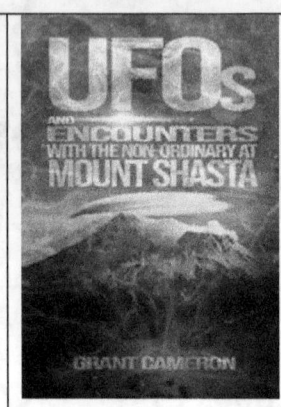
UFOs, Area 51 and Government Informants: Revised	The Portals and UFOs of Mount Shasta	UFOs and Encounters with the Non-Ordinary at Mount Shasta
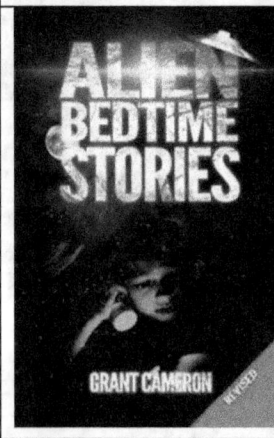	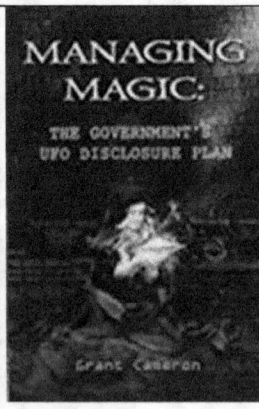	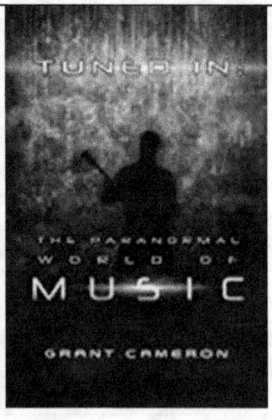
Alien Bedtime Stories Revised	Managing Magic: The Government's UFO Disclosure Plan	Tuned In: The Paranormal World of Music

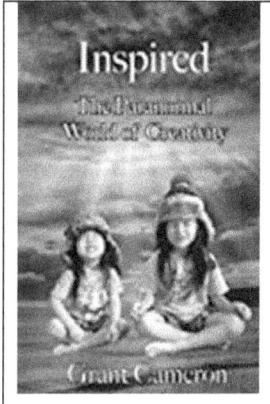	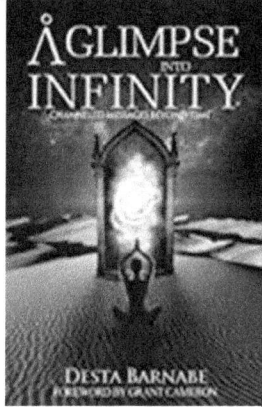	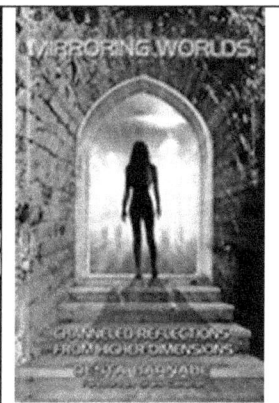
Inspired: The Paranormal World of Creativity	A Glimpse into Infinity: Channeled Messages	Mirroring Worlds: Channeled Messages

Amazon links:

https://www.amazon.com/s?k=grant+cameron&i=stripbooks&ref=nb_sb_noss_2

https://www.amazon.com/s?k=DESTA+BARNABE&i=stripbooks&ref=nb_sb_noss_2

Endnotes

1 MAPS Podcast Episode #6, "Ralph Metzner, A Life Lived in Expanded Consciousness," April 24, 2017. April 24, 2017

2 The Psychedelic Experience: A Manual Based on The Tibetan Book of the Dead, by Timothy Leary, Ralph Metzer and Richard Alpert. 1964, Zihuatanejo Project in Zihuatanejo, Mexico.

3 The Tim Ferriss Podcast Show #365 Michael Pollan.

4 Jim Fadiman on Psychedelics, MAPS Presentation, May 26, 2013, https://maps.org/news/media/4814-jim-fadiman-on-psychedelics-2

5 "Michael Pollan - Psychedelics and How to Change Your Mind | Bioneers," https://www.youtube.com/watch?v=5DrM90dg5t4

6 Alan Watts Quotes, https://www.goodreads.com/quotes/6639601-if-you-get-the-message-hang-up-the-phone-for

7 Eben Alexander, "Proof of Heaven," page 70.

8 Mercedes Sosa, "Gracias a la vida," https://www.youtube.com/watch?v=HcLQSKW0B3U

9 Frederick S. Barrett1 and Roland R. Griffiths, "Classic Hallucinogens and Mystical Experiences: Phenomenology and Neural Correlates,"https://www.ncbi.nlm.nih.gov/pmc/articles/PMC6707356/

1010 Seema Patel and Arun Goyal " developments in mushrooms as anti-cancer therapeutics: a review," https://www.ncbi.nlm.nih.gov/pmc/articles/PMC3339609/

11 "Terence Mckenna - Science Needed One Free Miracle, Humbleness," https://www.youtube.com/watch?v=i1q0CRY-X00&feature=share&fbclid=IwAR0iMA1hox9vPwAw8AOce8B34YOAlsaWLSU310Sk9kVGEXS4akZCAmh8IO4

12 Mateo Sol, "9 Signs You've Had a Mystical Experience," https://lonerwolf.com/mystical-experience/

13 Roland R. Griffiths, William A. Richards, Matthew W. Johnson, Una D. McCann, and Robert Jesse, "Mystical-type experiences occasioned by psilocybin mediate the attribution of personal meaning and spiritual significance 14 months later," https://www.ncbi.nlm.nih.gov/pmc/articles/PMC3050654/

14 "Joe Rogan Experience #1121 - Michael Pollan,"
https://www.youtube.com/watch?v=tz4CrWE_P0g
15 Ryan Kristobak, "Science Says This Playlist is a Must-Listen While Tripping on Mushrooms," https://theculturetrip.com/north-america/usa/articles/science-says-you-should-listen-to-this-music-while-tripping-on-mushrooms/
16 "LSD enhances the emotional response to music,"
https://www.researchgate.net/publication/280883331_LSD_enhances_the_emotional_response_to_music
17 Tim Ferriss Podcast Radio interview with Michael Pollan #365
18 Eric Dolan, "Study: 'Bad trips' from magic mushrooms often result in an improved sense of personal well-being,"
https://www.psypost.org/2016/08/study-bad-trips-from-magic-mushrooms-often-result-in-an-improved-sense-of-personal-well-being-44684
19 Journal of Pharmacology, "Cessation and reduction in alcohol consumption and misuse after psychedelic use,"
https://journals.sagepub.com/doi/abs/10.1177/0269881119845793
20 https://psychedelicreview.com/study-confirms-the-role-of-the-5-ht2a-receptor-in-the-psilocybin-psychedelic-experience/
21 The DMN is large-scale brain network primarily composed of the medial prefrontal cortex, posterior cingulate cortex/precuneus and angular gyrus.
22 Tanas, R.: The Passion of the Western Mind: Understanding the Ideas that Have Shaped Our World View. Ballantine Books, New York (1991)
23 Ten Laws with East Forest Podcast, "Dr. Robin Carhart-Harris interview Science of the Soul (#104)"
24 Richards, W. (2015). Sacred knowledge: psychedelics and religious experiences (Columbia University Press), Page 14-15.
25 " Psychedelics and the UFO/Et Experience,"
https://thetruthhides.wordpress.com/2013/09/23/psychedelics-and-the-ufoet-experience/
26 Beckley Foundation, "New evidence for a central role of music in psychedelic therapy,"
https://www.beckleyfoundation.org/2018/02/08/new-evidence-for-a-central-role-of-music-in-psychedelic-therapy/
27 The Anesteiologist feel the Sting, The Psilocybin Chronicles," October 6, 2019
28 Maps Podcast, Episode 20 – Dr. Williams Richards. MAPS Podcast Episode #6, "Ralph Metzner, A Life Lived in Expanded Consciousness," April 24, 2017. April 24, 2017.

29 Beckley Foundation, "New evidence for a central role of music in psychedelic therapy," https://www.beckleyfoundation.org/2018/02/08/new-evidence-for-a-central-role-of-music-in-psychedelic-therapy/

30 , Matthew W Johnson, Matthew W Johnson, , William A Richards, Brian D Richards, Robert Jesse, Katherine A MacLean, Frederick S Barrett, Mary P Cosimano, Maggie A Klinedinst, 'Psilocybin-occasioned mystical-type experience in combination with meditation and other spiritual practices produces enduring positive changes in psychological functioning and in trait measures of prosocial attitudes and behaviors," https://journals.sagepub.com/doi/full/10.1177/0269881117731279

31 Irving Kirsch ,"Antidepressants and the Placebo Effect," https://www.ncbi.nlm.nih.gov/pmc/articles/PMC4172306/

32 "Gender and Crime - Differences Between Male And Female Offending Patterns - Categories, Women, Females, and Males" - JRank Articles https://law.jrank.org/pages/1250/Gender-Crime-Differences-between-male-female-offending-patterns.html#ixzz6eCA7Fcy5

33 Communications Biology, "An improved neuroanatomical model of the default-mode network reconciles previous neuroimaging and neuropathological findings," https://www.nature.com/articles/s42003-019-0611-3

34 London Real Podcast, "What is the ego death& How does it change your Psychedelic Experience: Dennis McKenna," March 6, 2020.

35 Brian Robinson, "Brain Scientist Witnesses Her Own Stroke, Shares Tips On Life And Career," https://www.forbes.com/sites/bryanrobinson/2020/03/07/brain-scientist-witnesses-her-own-stroke-shares-tips-on-life-and-career/#75dbfde63949

36 Ibid.

37 Paul Ridden "Johns Hopkins study finds Psilocybin dosage 'sweet spot' for positive and lasting effects," https://newatlas.com/johns-hopkins-psilocybin-study-finds-optimum-beneficial-dosage/18981/

38 Ibid.

39 MAPS Podcast Episode #6, "Ralph Metzner, A Life Lived in Expanded Consciousness," April 24, 2017. April 24, 2017

40 "The Tim Ferriss Show Transcripts: Stan Grof (#347)," November 22, 2018, https://tim.blog/2018/11/22/the-tim-ferriss-show-transcripts-stan-grof/

41 "Joe Rogan Experience #1121 - Michael Pollan," https://www.youtube.com/watch?v=tz4CrWE_P0g

42 Braincast Podcast, "Illegal Drugs as Treatments in Psychiatry with Professor David Nutt."

43 Weird Wonderful Stories Podcast, "EP 68 Joong NDE Research Foundation."

44 My stroke of insight | Jill Bolte Taylor, https://www.youtube.com/watch?v=UyyjU8fzEYU

45 Oprah's SuperSoul Conversations - Dr. Jill Bolte Taylor "My Stroke of Insight" https://www.youtube.com/watch?v=yoclraXul4E

46 Brian Frank, "Scientists studying psychoactive drugs accidentally proved the self is an illusion," https://qz.com/1196408/scientists-studying-psilocybin-accidentally-proved-the-self-is-an-illusion/

47 "Psilocybin for treatment-resistant depression: fMRI-measured brain mechanisms," https://www.beckleyfoundation.org/resource/psilocybin-for-treatment-resistant-depression-fmri-measured-brain-mechanisms/

48 "Amanda Feilding - The Beckley Foundation's Scientific Programme," https://www.youtube.com/watch?v=g00e5Yimzh8

49 Aldous Huxley quotes," https://www.goodreads.com/work/quotes/23668205-the-doors-of-perception

50 Shavia Love, "LSD Changes Something About The Way You Perceive Time," https://www.vice.com/en_us/article/j5zd7p/lsd-changes-something-about-the-way-you-perceive-time

51 Keynote address: Perception, Illusion, and Truth | Donald Hoffman, https://www.youtube.com/watch?v=mgYoohATits

52 "Edgar Mitchell Quotes," https://www.goodreads.com/author/quotes/301350.Edgar_D_Mitchell

53 Michael Pollan - Psychedelics and How to Change Your Mind | Bioneers," https://www.youtube.com/watch?v=5DrM90dg5t4&list=PLzUs2NvAQs5_G2fSp85hxv82s-QTa59RL&index=130

54 Katya Kowalski, "Connectivity to Nature on Psychedelics," https://medium.com/@katya398/connectivity-to-nature-on-psychedelics-1b3d831d5e14

55 Tessa Love, "How LSD May Facilitate Communing With Nature: Researchers are finding evidence that hippies may have been onto something," https://elemental.medium.com/how-lsd-may-facilitate-communing-with-nature-de5d1004077a

56 "Eminent scientists reject the supernatural: a survey of the Fellows of the Royal Society," https://evolution-outreach.biomedcentral.com/articles/10.1186/1936-6434-6-33

57 "Survey of entity encounter experiences occasioned by inhaled N,N-dimethyltryptamine: Phenomenology, interpretation, and enduring effects,"
https://journals.sagepub.com/doi/full/10.1177/0269881120916143?fbcli
d=IwAR3Oar4JUAqdpslWhCvLPqoEKKAVCE_iRAi8pMndSbQBbflDEy
GsiuMliLg&
58 ATHEISTS FOUND "GOD" OR "ULTIMATE REALITY" AFTER
TAKING   PSYCHEDELIC   DRUGS,
https://www.inverse.com/article/55228-atheists-stopped-being-
atheists-after-taking-psychedelics
59 Conversations with the Mind Podcast, "Episode 61 – Dr. James Fadiman: The Godfather of Microdosing Psychedelics."
60 Brian Prank, "Scientists studying psychoactive drugs accidentally proved the self is an illusion," https://qz.com/1196408/scientists-
studying-psilocybin-accidentally-proved-the-self-is-an-illusion/
61 "The Definition and Concept of Maya in Hinduism,"
https://www.hinduwebsite.com/hinduism/essays/maya.asp
62 https://www.brainyquote.com/authors/niels-bohr-quotes
63 "DMT Models the Near-Death Experience,"
https://www.frontiersin.org/articles/10.3389/fpsyg.2018.01424/full
64 "Neural correlates of the psychedelic state as determined by fMRI studies with psilocybin,"
https://www.ncbi.nlm.nih.gov/pmc/articles/PMC3277566/
65 Glenn F. Chesnut, " Father Ed Dowling: Bill Wilson's Sponsor," Glenn F. Chesnut
66 E. Kurtz, " Drugs and the Spiritual: Bill W. takes LSD,"
http://www.williamwhitepapers.com/pr/1989%20Bill%20W%20takes%
20LSD.pdf
67 The Systemic Psychedelic, "Dr. Rich Strassman on Corona, Creativity and Psychedelics as Super Placebos April 27, 2020
68 Earth Ancients Podcast, "Rich Strassman: DMT and the Soul of Prophecy."
69 Rick Stausman, "The Spirit Molecule,"
https://files.meetup.com/17628282/DMT-The-spirit-molecule.pdf
70 "William James on Consciousness and the Four Features of Transcendent Experiences,"
https://www.brainpickings.org/2018/06/04/william-james-varieties-
consciousness/
71 I came to believe this as I worked as a bartender at the Faculty Club at the University of Manitoba for a number of years. In that position I dealt with hundreds of professors, lecturers, deans, vice-presidents, and

presidents. I had long UFO discussions with three faculty deans, and after many debates with the dean of plant science I realized that he knew nothing about UFOs. It was an ah-hah moment for me.

72 "Shoomery Magic Mushrooms Demystified,"
https://www.shroomery.org/6255/Trip-Reports
73 Kilindi Iyi - High-Dose Mushrooms Beyond the Threshold,
https://www.youtube.com/watch?v=ejdKeghBhNs